LINDSAY WAGNER'S
NEW BEAUTY

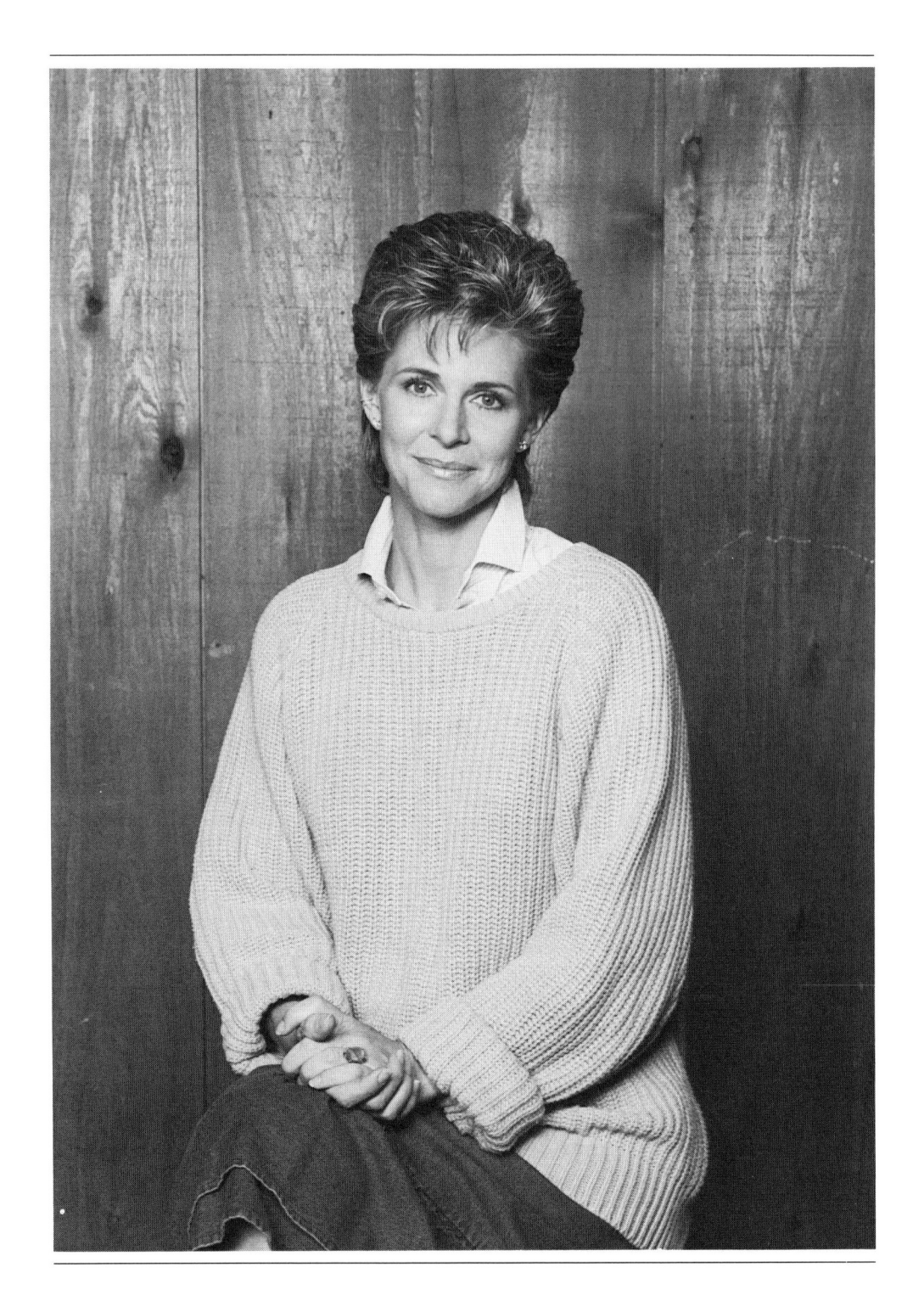

LINDSAY WAGNER'S NEW BEAUTY
THE ACUPRESSURE FACELIFT

BY LINDSAY WAGNER
AND ROBERT M. KLEIN

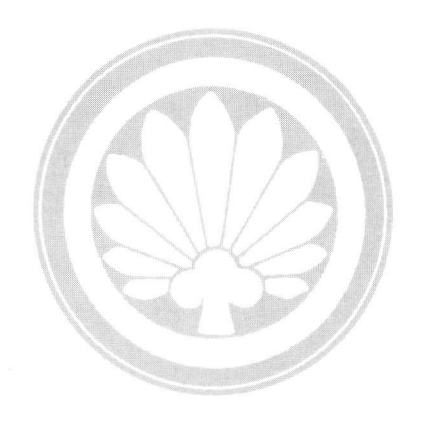

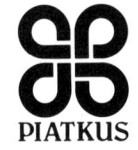

PIATKUS

This book is not intended in any way whatsoever to serve as a manual for self-treatment of medical problems. Any such problems should be brought to the attention of the reader's physician. Any application of the ideas and information contained herein is done so solely at the discretion and risk of the reader.

Copyright © 1987 by Lindsay Wagner/Wagner Ball Productions, Inc., and Robert M. Klein
Photographs copyright © 1986 by Peter Kredenser/Shooting Star

First published in Great Britain in 1988 by Judy Piatkus (Publishers) Ltd of 5 Windmill Street, London W1

British Library Cataloguing in Publication Data
Wagner, Lindsay
 The 30-day natural facelift programme:
 using the acupressure massage technique.
 1. Beauty care. Use of Shiatzu
 I. Title II. Klein, Robert M.
 646.7'2

 ISBN 0-86188-774-3
 ISBN 0-86188-779-4 Pbk

Printed and bound in Great Britain by Butler & Tanner Ltd, Frome, Somerset

To my sons, Alex Nathan and Dorian Henry

ACKNOWLEDGMENTS

LINDSAY WAGNER: I want to thank Verrel Reed and Dr. William Hornaday for helping to open my eyes, and Gladys McGarey and Robert Lorenz for helping me to see.

BOB KLEIN: This book has come about with the inspiration and help of many—Gim Shek Ju, the master acupuncturist, who opened his door and then his knowledge to me; my good friends Dr. Marshall Ho'o and to H. Y. Lee, who have unfolded great knowledge about Oriental healing and martial arts for Western understanding; Marcia Dale Weiss, who helped open so many inner doors; Dr. Gary Richwald, always an inspiration with his extraordinary medical skills; Iona Teeguarden, a master teacher and practitioner of acupressure; Marty Zucker, whose journalistic and editing skills honed this book into final shape; Claire and Jake, for so much loving family support during this book project; and to the memory of Justine, whose sweet spirit lives on within me.

CONTENTS

PART I THE NATURAL NO-SURGERY FACELIFT

    It Really Goes to Work Fast
        by Lindsay Wagner   13
    What is the Acupressure Facelift All About?
        by Robert M. Klein   21
    Acupressure versus Surgical Facelift   31

PART II HOW TO GIVE YOURSELF THE ACUPRESSURE FACELIFT

    Get Ready . . .   37
    . . . Go!   45
    Questions and Answers   85

PART III LINDSAY WAGNER'S TOTAL APPROACH TO BEAUTY

    Getting Your Body and Head behind Your Face   99
    Eating for Better Health, Energy, and Beauty   103
    Rest, Relaxation, and Stress   117
    Beauty Tips   123
    Some Parting Words   131

PART IV APPENDIXES

Appendix A: Vitamins	134
Appendix B: Minerals	137
Appendix C: Food Combinations	140

PART I

THE NATURAL NO-SURGERY FACELIFT

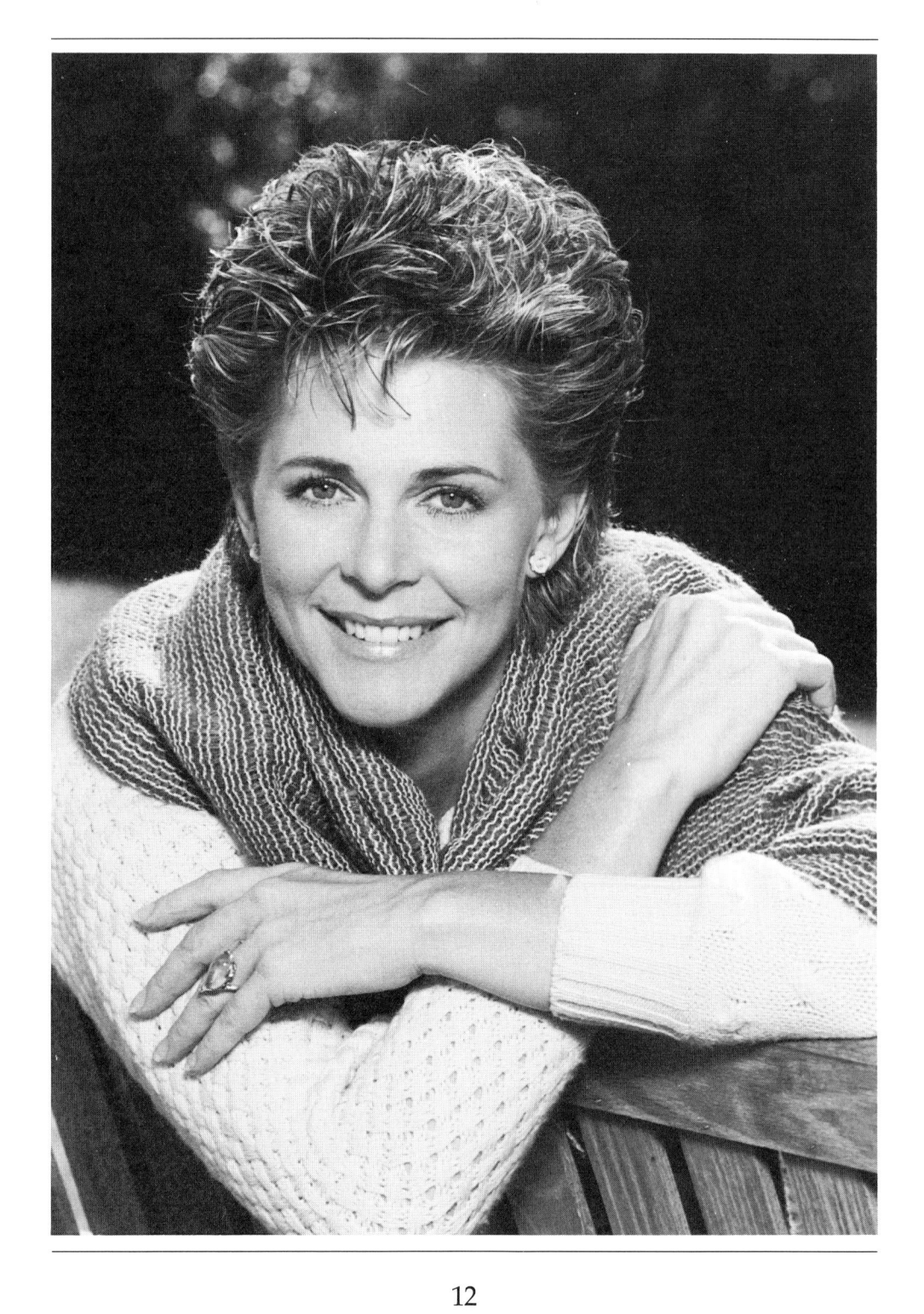

IT REALLY GOES TO WORK FAST

BY LINDSAY WAGNER

Okay, I can hear what you're thinking already. . . . Who needs another beauty book by another celebrity, with her cheekbones, straight teeth, and hair that would look good even if it had been cut with hedge clippers—who also spends half of her waking hours in front of a mirror in order to look that way? I promise you, this is not one of those books! This comes from someone who, just a short time ago, considered a quick scrub with clear soap and a dash out the door a complete beauty treatment.

I have always felt that what's inside is what one should keep working on, and, that if you are content, the outside will reflect it. Well, that's true in part. But, alas, let me also tell you that lately I have discovered some disturbing news: Galileo was right. Gravity is a reality and it *does* affect *all* bodies; it does not discriminate. Actors can least afford to wake up one morning and find all parts heading south! So . . . since my chosen profession requires me to keep the chassis together and the paint looking new, further measures were called for.

I hate the idea of plastic surgery. Although it does provide a new

Trivial Pursuit question for your friends, ("Who do you suppose did the job?"), it is risky, invasive, and expensive. I am not saying it doesn't work; but, unless you are being mistaken for a Shar Pei, it should only be considered as a last resort.

I want to tell you about something very exciting that you can do for yourself. It is a *natural* facelift you can do at home or even on the job. It goes to work on wrinkles and those wonderful *laugh* lines (as we choose to call them); it firms up the sags and bags and brings a vibrant new glow to your face. Not only does it improve your looks, it also relaxes you and makes you feel better. It does not require you to buy any expensive equipment. All you need are your hands and fifteen or twenty minutes daily.

This technique has been taught to men and women of all ages and from all walks of life—with great success. It is a simple method that anyone of you can learn in minutes (as long as you can still find your face with your hands). The technique is called the Acupressure Facelift. No, I didn't say "acupuncture," so put the knitting needles back in the drawer.

When the Acupressure Facelift first came to my attention, I was familiar enough with the word *acupressure* from my interest in holistic medicine and fitness. I had used general acupressure treatments for physical toning and shaping, but I did not know how it could be applied to a facelift.

The word *acupressure* refers to a system of massage, or healing pressure, applied to points on the body by the fingers. (Just to make sure we all understand which is which, acu*puncture* uses needles, acu*pressure* uses the fingers.) Both acupuncture and acupressure are forms of ancient Oriental healing arts that were practiced on the faces of

Chinese emperors and empresses thousands of years ago. But the good news is . . . it works equally well on the overworked people of the eighties!

I became excited about the idea of a "hands on" facelift that people could do for themselves. It fit in with my attitude toward general health; one should take responsibility for one's own health; surgery should be avoided unless it is absolutely necessary and then, only when all other forms of treatment are exhausted. The natural facelift described in this book can give each of you the satisfying opportunity for better health and beauty in your lifetime.

When Bob Klein first offered to teach me the method, I was just leaving for London to do a talk show. I grabbed the closest guinea pig available, my business partner, who just happens to be my mother. She could be working with it during my absence. She made the perfect subject, for two reasons: (1) she is difficult to convince and (2) she admits to having lost the war against gravity.

When I returned from London, in just two short weeks, the changes I observed in my mother were significant: I immediately noticed that the lines around her mouth had become considerably less pronounced. They were perhaps *half* of what they had been before! *And* she seemed very relaxed (until I told her what the trip cost!). I told her that I thought the method was working wonders. Mother's comments were somewhat cautious. She, too, thought the lines were softening, but she was afraid to be more enthusiastic, she wasn't sure if her eyesight was going, or if there had really been some genuine changes.

But I was convinced and immediately decided to learn the method.

I recall vividly the first time I tried the process. It was a stressful time for me: long hours on preproduction of a TV movie called *Child's Cry* (which called for a lot of research at a center for child abuse), in addition to my responsibilities at home as a mother of an active three-year-old. By the time I finished the Acupressure Facelift that day, the natural color was back in my face. I felt surprisingly relaxed and rejuvenated.

Encouraged, I started to apply the technique on a daily basis. At first, I tried doing it in the morning before work, but not being the most organized person in the world, too many times I found myself rushing out the door, orange juice in one hand and a script in the other. The good news is that I soon realized I could do it during shooting lulls on location, with the same pleasant results! One of the joys of this method is that, once you learn it, you can do it anywhere, anytime. After just seven days, the texture of my skin seemed to have undergone a dramatic softening. I performed the procedure daily for a month and, each time, it felt as though I had been given a facial. I began to notice a definite improvement in the lines around my eyes and elsewhere on my face.

I don't know about you, but there are certain areas of my face that have always demanded extra attention. During a filming, they required more frequent application of makeup. Now I am finding that my makeup is staying on more uniformly, and for longer periods of time. Hallie Smith-Simmons, my makeup artist, is delighted with this welcome change: Her work has been cut in half!

Perhaps the ultimate testimonial came when I visited Soshin, a very talented Japanese lady in Santa Monica who gives me facials from time to time. Usually, she would scowl and tell me I had stayed away too long. She happily remarked that my skin looked great! When someone who works on your face at close range makes such a positive observation, you know something good is happening.

And it is still happening: Sometimes when I'm working, tension accumulates and it shows in my face. During the filming of *Child's Cry*, I was faced with a good deal of emotional and stressful experiences, due to the nature of the subject. I was constantly seeing things that were painful to me, and I found myself becoming tense and drawn. I *needed* to relax; the emotional benefits of an acupressure facial massage were of immense help.

Speaking of children and the need to relax, quite often I come home after a twelve-hour workday only to find that my four-year-old has mistaken me for Darth Vadar. He ambushes me with a light saber and I am not expected to surrender easily. Sometimes the battle goes on for hours. Once he's in bed, in a galaxy far, far away, I can sit by the fire, listen to soft music, and massage away the tension in my face. I value the technique for its immediate benefits, but the long-range effects also prove that, if you feel better, you look better.

Fine. So now you want to know just how long and how often you have to do this. You know as well as I do that the beginning of any new project requires the most effort. To get started, you should plan to use the method daily and to devote approximately twenty minutes to it. After the first month of daily applications, when you have begun to see the results you want, I would say you could then cut back to three or four times a week—that should be fine for maintaining optimal facial ''shape.'' In the following chapters you will learn with both pictures and words all about this simple and natural nonsurgical facelift. I will show you how to do the method yourself. It won't take long before you have become an expert. You will feel something exciting happening the very first time. To *see* results quickly, though, you must follow the instructions carefully and practice the program as laid out.

In no time at all, you will have more circulation in and around your face, bringing with it a youthful luster, and, as the tissue beneath your skin becomes vitalized and fills out, your laugh lines will stop laughing and the crinkles around your mouth will start to fade.

Aside from repairing the footprints of time, acupressure is also an insurance program for people in their twenties. Trust me, with the exception of Dick Clark, no one is going to look twenty forever. The rest of us will have to be grateful for this technique, which slows down facial aging and retards the slings and arrows of outrageous fortune . . . *we're talking preventive maintenance here*!

If you believe, as many do these days, that exercise is necessary to maintain a healthy body and mind, just think of the Acupressure Facelift as the fitness program for your face. (And you won't need to bounce around in designer outfits to get it in shape either.) Isn't it funny how we exercise our bodies and elaborately cover them up, while we walk around with our sagging faces exposed to the world?

Congratulations! By the time you have finished this program, your face will be as fit as your figure. One last thing: I have written a section on my ideas about a total approach to beauty. I will be talking about food, rest, relaxation, how I deal with stress, and aspects of one's life-style that I feel contribute to well-being in general.

Now that I have said something about how I feel about the Acupressure Facelift and what it has done for me, I will let Bob Klein tell you about just *why* it works.

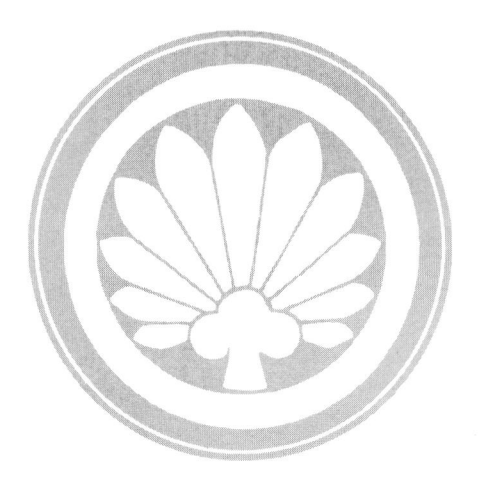

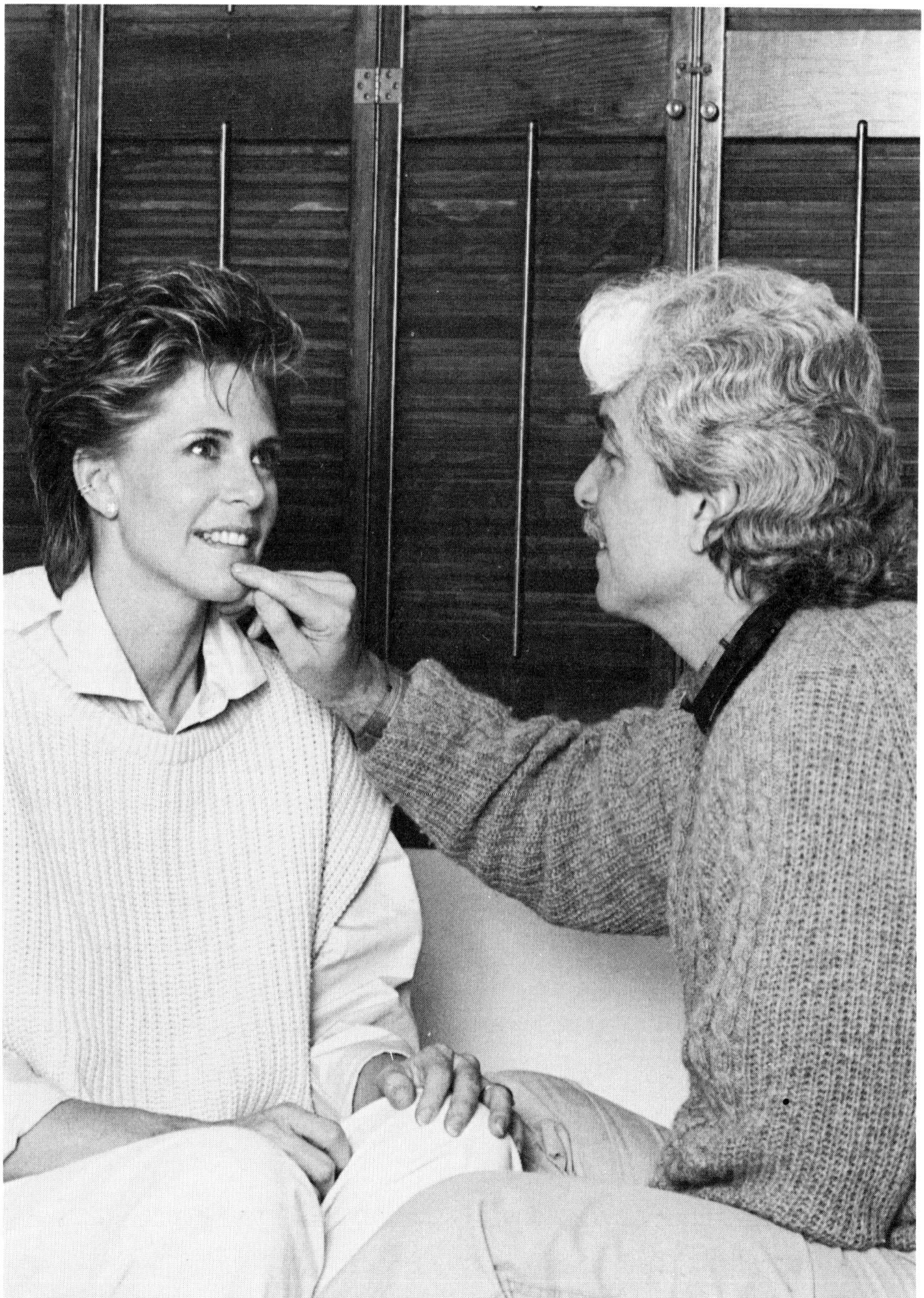

WHAT IS THE ACUPRESSURE FACELIFT ALL ABOUT?

BY ROBERT M. KLEIN

Since 1975 I have been teaching the Acupressure Facelift. The results have been so outstanding that I wanted to reach as large an audience as possible, to shout it from the rooftops and let the whole world know about and benefit from it. That's why Lindsay and I have written this book and filmed a videotape.

I learned about the technique from a great Chinese master—Gim Shek Ju—under whom I studied acupuncture for four years. On my own, I researched and learned more about the procedure; later, as a health counselor working under medical doctors in the Los Angeles area, I was able to teach the procedure to many individuals.

The first person I taught was myself, and the first thing I noticed was that I felt better. Then I began to notice that I looked better. Thinking that I might simply be seeing something I was predisposed to seeing, I just kept my mouth shut and kept at it.

Changes continued to come. Whenever I did the procedure I felt absolutely relaxed afterward. Stress lines in my face softened, and my face seemed to radiate new vigor. I really did start to look and feel different—and all for the better. When people started to make comments and ask what I was doing, I then felt confident enough to start sharing the information.

From the start, the results were positive and immediate. I taught politicians, business people, some very well known celebrities—people in all walks of life, both men and women of all ages.

They would come back after a week and use words like "amazing," "fantastic," and "wonderful." Consistently, they said that they looked and felt better. The feedback from people in show business was particularly encouraging to me. The very nature of this work puts critical importance on one's appearance.

After she had been doing the facial massage for about a month, one well-known actress told me she had been "accused" of having a surgical facelift. She had been motivated to try the technique because she was no longer being offered her usual roles as a young innocent woman, and instead was being cast as a mother. After using the technique regularly, she was cast in roles more suitable for her age.

ROOTS IN ANTIQUITY

This wonderful self-help facial treatment has its roots in antiquity, in the profound wisdom that comes from ancient medical knowledge and teachings. Thousands of years ago, medical scholars in Asia mapped out a system or network of bodily energy. The Chinese called it *chi*; the Japanese name for it is *ki*. Knowledge of this energy system forms the basis of acupuncture.

You can think of the system as the "body's battery pack." It is an invisible grid of energy channels throughout the body that really run the machinery; it is the life-force that allows the blood and lymph to flow and the muscles to work. It maintains harmony and balance among the organs and working parts, and it energizes the cells. We cannot physically see this energy flow, but science is able to measure it electronically.

Acupuncture is an ancient and well-established healing art used for the treatment of illnesses, the relief of pain, and for the general balancing of bodily energy. It gained popularity in the United States following President Nixon's visit to China in the early 1970s.

In acupuncture fine needles are gently inserted at various points in the body to stimulate or sedate the flow of energy. There are literally hundreds of these "acupuncture points" on the body, located along certain energy pathways known as "meridians." These meridians run from the top of the head to the tips of the toes. Each one corresponds directly to certain vital organs of the body.

These acupuncture points are cup shaped. You can feel them by grazing your fingertips lightly over an area until you feel a slight depression just below the surface of the skin. An easy one to find is on your hands where your thumb and forefinger join. This acupuncture point is related to the function of the large intestine and to the flow of energy to the face.

When any of these acupuncture points are blocked or congested, the result is "unwellness." The flow of energy throughout the body is affected and put in imbalance. Because of the interconnection of the meridians, problems can appear in seemingly unrelated parts of the body.

Points can be blocked or congested from a variety of causes, including the following:

- External trauma, such as a blow to the body

- Internal trauma, such as an illness

- Stress and tension; pressure at home or work

- Air, water, and noise pollution

- Poor diets of highly processed, highly chemicalized, and highly unnatural food

- The harsh, drying effect on the skin of ultraviolet light; the detrimental radiation from fluorescent lights, television tubes, or video display terminals

Clearly, our bodies are under constant siege from the elements—both inside and outside us. The long-term effect of life's stresses eventually have to show up somewhere on the body; it seems that the face is one of the first places.

At a subtle level, many of the acupuncture points on the face regularly become blocked or congested. The circulation of energy to the facial tissue and muscles is impaired, causing degeneration and sagging. Among the telltale signs are these: The skin begins to dry out, blotches of discoloration appear, muscles lose their tone, cheeks and jowls start to sag, and wrinkles spread and deepen at a frightening pace. We look harder, older than our years.

ACUPUNCTURE AND ACUPRESSURE

Up to now I have been speaking about acupuncture points. Just where does acupressure come in and what's the difference between the two?

Acupressure is based on the same system of points and meridians as acupuncture. Instead of inserting needles, however, you simply massage these points with the tips of your fingers. A warmth is created, which converts into a minute electrical charge. This charge feeds the muscles, nerves, and lymphatic system, clearing the meridians that are blocked.

When you start to use the acupressure technique Lindsay and I will be teaching you, you will increase the circulation of blood and energy within your face. Not only will you start to feel better but the lines in your face will soften and you will actually look younger. You will experience fresh color in your face. You will radiate with a healthy glow.

It is important to understand that neither acupuncture nor acupressure are cures in and of themselves. What both techniques do is facilitate the body's own natural impulse toward balance. When internal energy is flowing easily and well, the body's systems operate harmoniously with one another. Healing is enhanced. The result is better health.

In ancient times, Oriental rulers received daily treatments from their own private acupuncturists. Great emphasis was placed on preventing disease. This, in fact, was regarded as the highest expression of

Chinese medicine. Doctors were paid to keep you healthy; when you fell ill, payment was withheld.

Treatment for the royal ladies in those days included a fingertip massage of the acupuncture points on the face. That is where the Acupressure Facelift concept began. It was designed to retard the signs of aging, to keep the skin youthful and glowing, and to keep the facial muscles toned, in addition to giving benefit to other parts of the body.

What makes the Acupressure Facelift so special is that it is a treatment you can give yourself each and every day. You do not have to be the emperor's wife to afford it. You can do it for yourself . . . free of charge.

The Acupressure Facelift takes up just fifteen to twenty minutes of your day, just once a day for one month. Afterward you can go to two or three times a week. Within this short time you will bring back beauty to your face and better health and efficiency to your body through more balanced energy. It is this energy flow that will help you to achieve a facelift that is safer, more natural looking and longer-lasting than any superimposed by surgery.

THE BENEFITS GO BEYOND THE FACE

The face is a veritable "road map" of points and meridians that, in fact, relate to all the parts of the body. When you stimulate and unblock some of these points, as you will be doing in the facial massage, you will be rejuvenating tired tissue with new energy and more nutrition, but you also may be doing some widespread good for yourself.

You will be stimulating points on your face that have acupuncture relationships to headaches, digestion, and circulation; to the sinuses, kidneys, lungs, heart, and intestines. Do not be surprised if you start feeling better all over.

In promoting this technique Lindsay and I occasionally hear from reporters who have written about the Acupressure Facelift and tried it themselves. Several have reported to us that headaches or digestion improved or that some minor physical problems cleared up. One woman reporter called us from the East Coast and said that, since starting the program, her constipation problem had cleared up! Was the connection possible? We told her it certainly was.

A politician who was running for public office was referred to me. He was rather skeptical about the idea of a natural facelift, yet he was willing to try it. He wanted to look better without undergoing surgery. Although he lost the election, he was a winner in the mirror. There were even some remarks in the press suggesting he had undergone some facial reconstruction. This same politician had suffered from some chronic digestive discomfort. After starting the program, he found that the problem abated. This effect could have resulted from the activation and clearance of key points in his face or simply from the relaxation brought about by doing the technique; perhaps it was a combination of both.

Please be aware, though, that we aren't making any medical claims for the massage, but it is just possible that good things might happen elsewhere in your body as you start to stimulate your facial energy channels. The points in your face are definitely connected to the rest of your body.

A short time after you start the program, your body will seem to ask for the massage. It wants the benefits, the healing fingers. It will ask, just as it asks you to respond to a sensation here or there elsewhere on the body, such as tension in the neck and shoulders. You recognize that sensation and immediately rub the area.

With the Acupressure Facelift technique, when you feel some tension on some part of your face, you will know exactly what to do. Such tension could be an early warning of eventual breakdown of localized circulation and tissue. Regard the signal. The fingertip massage we will be teaching you in this book is an answer to that signal. Use it as a tool. Anytime. For the rest of your life.

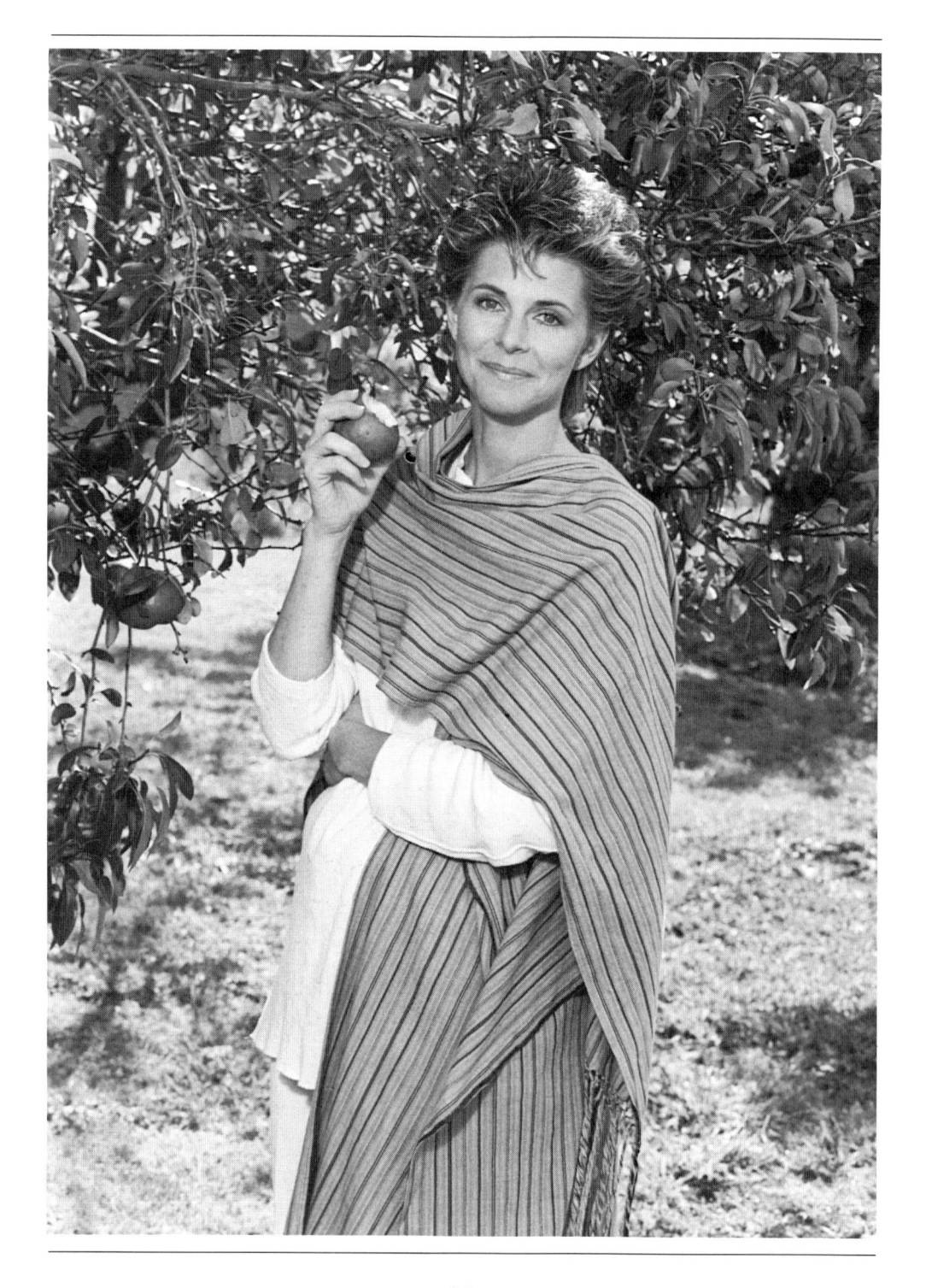

ACUPRESSURE VERSUS SURGICAL FACELIFT

How does all this compare to the regular facelift as we know it in Western society?

For practically everyone, the concept of a facelift conjures up the image and expectation of a surgical procedure that is going to restore beauty and youth to the face. That doesn't quite mesh with reality in most cases.

Plastic surgery does not stop the aging process. As plastic surgeons themselves admit, they may be able to turn back the clock some, but they cannot stop the ticking, nor can they make anyone look much younger than they are chronologically. A successful operation can make people look very well for their given age. They will look rested and rejuvenated; others will compliment them on how good they look, but that is as far as it goes. What's more, plastic surgery often changes the character of a person's face, creating an artificial image. It seems like more than just the lines are removed.

Dry and lackluster skin, lines, and sag are not just signs of a face getting older. They also represent neglect and stress. To attempt to deal with these signs exclusively through surgical removal is, in essence, to deny your body a chance to confront the problem itself in a more natural way. You are dealing with the effects and ignoring the causes.

With surgery, you may temporarily lose some lines, but your benefits are limited. Surgery will not restore life and vitality to your face. If you stop to think about it, in this procedure a surgeon is doing nothing more than basically stretching your skin over a layer of sagging and atrophied tissue.

The Acupressure Facelift deals with the skin and the supporting muscle tissue below it, and that is a *big* difference. It restores form and vitality to facial muscles that have gone soft due to lack of use and lack of circulation.

Here is a point of comparison: If you never exercise your arms, your biceps and triceps become flabby. The whole area will eventually sag. However, once you start exercising your arms, the tissue quickly firms up, and you have none of the unsightly sag. The same principle applies to your face.

A surgical facelift is not a one-shot procedure. It usually calls for tuck-ups and secondary facelifts anywhere from eighteen months to five years after the initial operation.

Impossible to ignore, too, is the cost factor. Surgical procedures are expensive. A plastic surgeon can sometimes work wonders on a face, but it may cost you an arm and a leg. You can pay up to ten thousand dollars for one facelift. (Payable in advance, please, since it is usually a purely cosmetic operation and not covered by medical insurance plans.)

Like any surgery (even a simple tooth extraction), conventional facelifts also carry a risk of complication. There is another factor to consider, too. No matter how skilled the physician, surgery intrudes upon, damages, and interrupts that network or system of bodily energy that we described earlier. Some delicate or subtle functions at other parts of the body can be affected when the face is operated on.

Conventional facelifts involve hospitalization, general anesthetic, bandages to wear after discharge, and facial discoloration. People usually "hide out," until all the annoying evidence has faded.

With the Acupressure Facelift there is none of this. No big expenditure. No risks. No hospitalization. No trauma to the body.

The Acupressure Facelift is totally natural. It's something you can do for yourself and by yourself. All you have to do is follow the simple directions in this book. Your only investment is the price of the book, a bit of time (just a few minutes really), and the energy it takes to give yourself a fingertip massage over your face.

If you follow the advice in this book, you may never need a surgical facelift. If you have been planning or seriously thinking about cosmetic surgery, just delay your decision and try this first. We think you will be surprised. For sure, you will look better and feel better.

PART II

HOW TO GIVE YOURSELF THE ACUPRESSURE FACELIFT

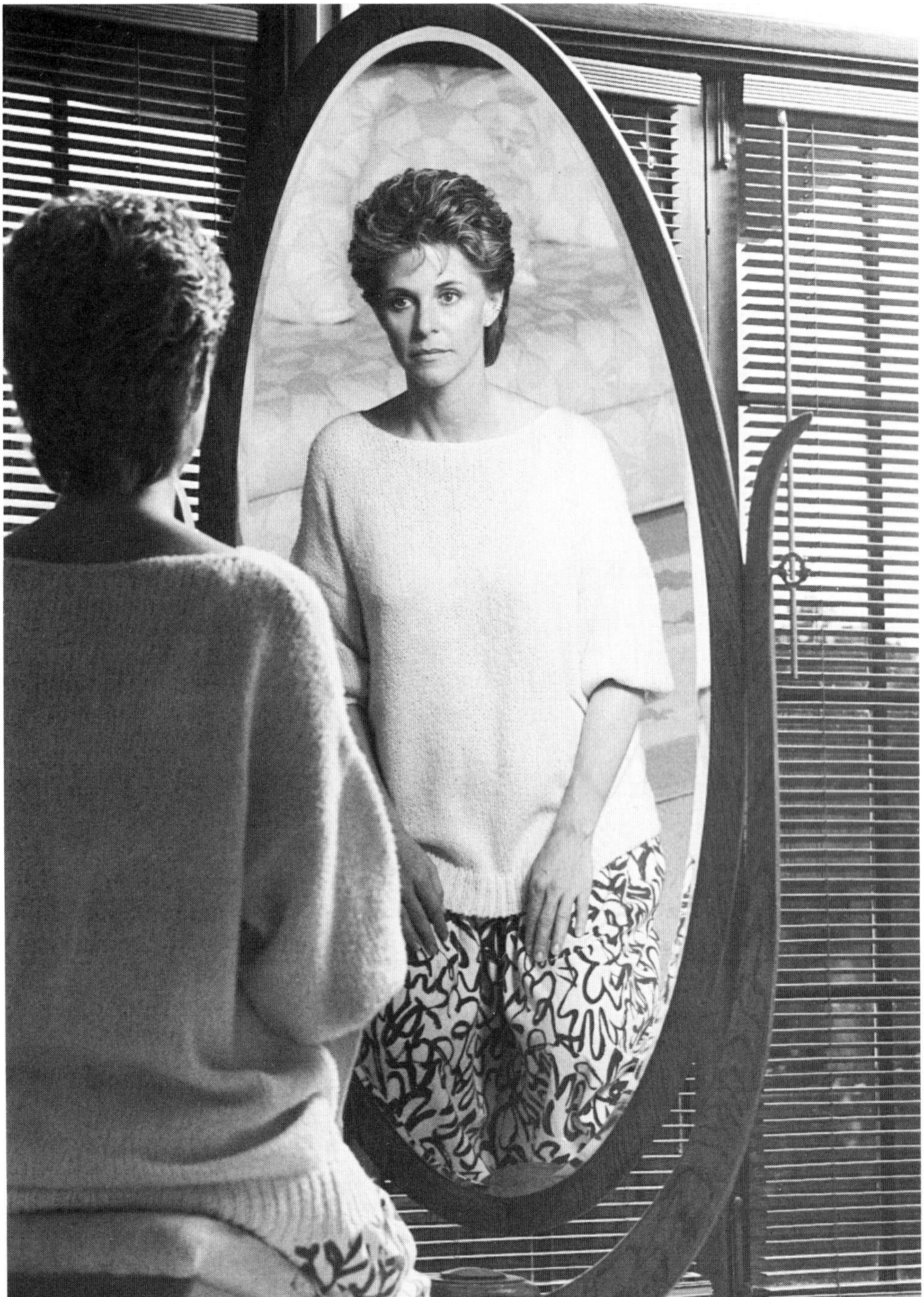

GET READY...

Now that you know what the Acupressure Facelift is all about and what it can do for you, let's get ready to do it.

Here is some start-up information that you will need to know.

For the first month—or thirty days—we recommend that you do the routine every day. Afterward, you can gear down to a maintenance program of two or three times a week. If you feel like it, of course, you can always do more.

By doing the massage every day for the first month you are really opening up an energy and circulation system that has most likely been working for a long time at a pretty tired level.

The meridians are like a fire hose. If the hose has nothing running through it, it is flat, full of snags, and kind of pressed together and dry. When water starts to flow through, it opens wider and wider. That is just what we want to do—open up the channels of energy.

The massage can be done at any time during the day. Make it convenient for yourself, but try to set aside those fifteen to twenty minutes when you will not have to rush and cut corners while doing the procedure. If you cut corners, you cut results.

Doing it in the morning is a wonderful way to start the day. If you normally exercise at that time and you can take the extra time, add the facial massage to your program. The new tone you see and the new energy you feel in your face will help give you a positive send-off for the day's activities.

Doing it in the evening is an equally satisfying way to unwind. You can combine it with some relaxation technique or energizing meditation, or do it while you have a "meeting" with yourself to go over the day's events or activities. Or just sit back and do it to your favorite music.

One New York woman tells us she does it sometimes on the subway ride either to or from work. On occasion, she says, her cotravelers will ask her what she is doing. When she explains, they sometimes start doing it themselves right there.

In other words, it doesn't matter when you do it. The point is just to do it.

In the very beginning, until you get familiar with the location of the points, use the illustrations in the next chapter to guide you through each massage step. It will not take long at all for you to learn them. You will be amazed at how easy the method is to do.

You will feel a slight depression at the site of most of the points. You may also feel some tenderness there. That's all right. That is another indication that you are on target.

Unless otherwise indicated, each of the points in the program should be massaged for about one minute. Whether you do a little more or a little less is not critical. You may want to look at a watch or clock in the beginning, but don't become obsessed about the amount of time. You will soon establish a smooth rhythm and pace of your own and you won't even glance at a watch.

Most of the points are bilateral; that is, located on both the right and left sides of your face. Unless otherwise directed, massage both points simultaneously with each hand.

Use just enough pressure to feel the point. Do not push hard enough to hurt. Just apply good, firm pressure.

Sometimes people have a tendency to push the face into the fingers. That can cause some tension and stiffness in the neck that way. The "style" we recommend is that you push the fingers into the face.

In the beginning your face might feel a little sore. It's a similar situation to when you begin an exercise program and activate unused muscles. Don't be alarmed at any residual tenderness; it will pass in a few days.

For this reason it's a good idea not to do the Acupressure Facelift more than once a day in the beginning. As with any new exercise, overdoing it can make the muscles sore. Just take it easy and follow the prescribed pace. The program is designed to bring you maximum results. Be patient and you will see results soon enough.

In addition to referring to the pictures, we suggest you also use a mirror at the start. Probably after doing it two or three times with a mirror you will be able to quickly zero in on each point. After a while, your fingers will locate them automatically. The procedure will eventually become so second nature to you that you will find yourself mindlessly massaging your face while you are at work, at a stoplight, talking on the phone, lying in bed, listening to music, or watching television.

> LINDSAY: *At any given time, when I am sitting, be it sitting on the set between shots or when I am nursing my baby or when I'm driving, I may find myself working a facial point automatically. And I won't be thinking which point it is I am working. My fingers often just seem to be responding to some subtle call from my body.*

Make yourself comfortable. You can do it sitting, standing, or lying down.

Check to see if your shoulders are tight and pulled up, which they might very well be at the end of a tense workday, for example. If they are, try to relax them by rolling them down, back, up, forward, and back down again. Then reverse the pattern. Rolling your shoulders like that can reduce tension. You can also roll your neck to the left and right a few times if you wish.

While you are massaging, try to breathe deeply and rhythmically. In through your nose. Out through your mouth. This will help keep you relaxed and energized, and it also increases the elimination of accumulated toxins through the lungs.

Try also to maintain a uniform tempo through the massaging of the points. Many people listen to music while they do the facelift procedure to help them maintain a constant tempo. Music produced on the Windham Hill label is particularly soothing and conducive to this meditative routine, although any relaxing music will do.

If you encounter a blemish or sore at some point along the way, avoid doing that particular point until the condition heals.

Do not let fear of breaking long fingernails stop you. There is another way to massage. Use your knuckles—bending and using the second joint on your fingers. Put that joint onto the point and massage that way. It works just as well as the fingertips. Some people alternate between fingertips and knuckles just for variety. If you are going to be using the knuckles, you may want to first find the point with your fingertip, since it is more sensitive. You can also use the knuckle method if your fingers get tired.

Please keep in mind that the total program and its overall effect is of great importance. Although we describe the localized benefits of each point, experience shows conclusively that these individual effects are multiplied when done within the context of the entire program. The whole is definitely greater than the sum of the parts.

For your information, we are providing the traditional Chinese names of the points and some of their healing attributes, as established in Oriental medicine. However, neither this nor any other information contained in the book is intended for the use of self-therapy. If you have any physical ailment, please consult a physician.

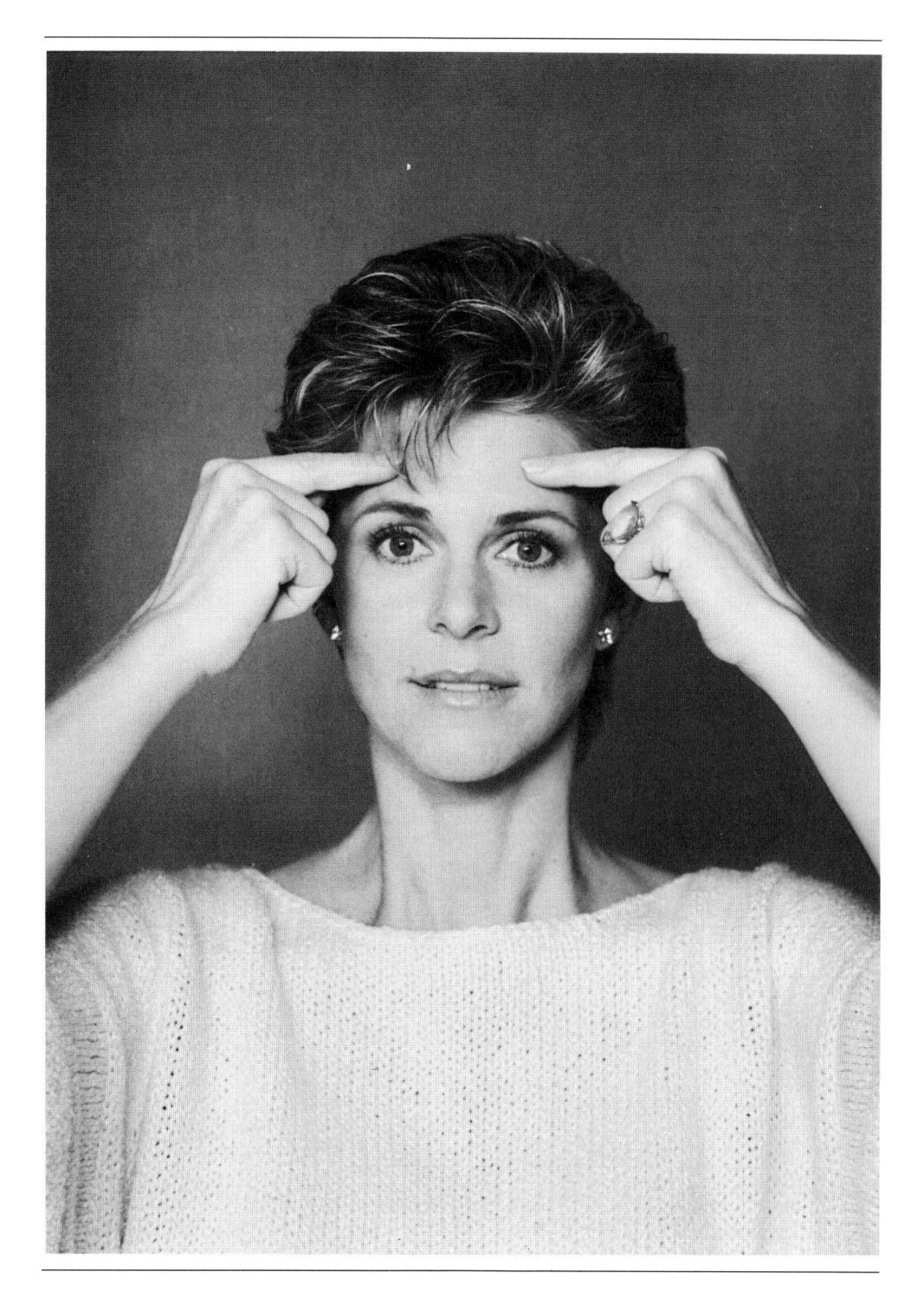

...GO!

LINDSAY: *OK. You're all set. Remember these key tips:*

- *Once a day for the first thirty days.*

- *Two or three times a week afterward. More, if you like.*

- *Don't overdo it in the beginning. Stick to the schedule.*

- *Relax. Make yourself comfortable. Try to maintain a relaxed and steady rhythm throughout the routine.*

- *Give yourself about one minute on each point, unless otherwise indicated.*

- *Apply firm pressure to the points with your fingers, hard enough to feel, but not hard enough to hurt.*

- *After you are finished, sit quietly for a few minutes. You will begin to feel the energy and increased circulation in your face. Feel your face come alive. You will be aware of the new vigor, health, and beauty in your face.*

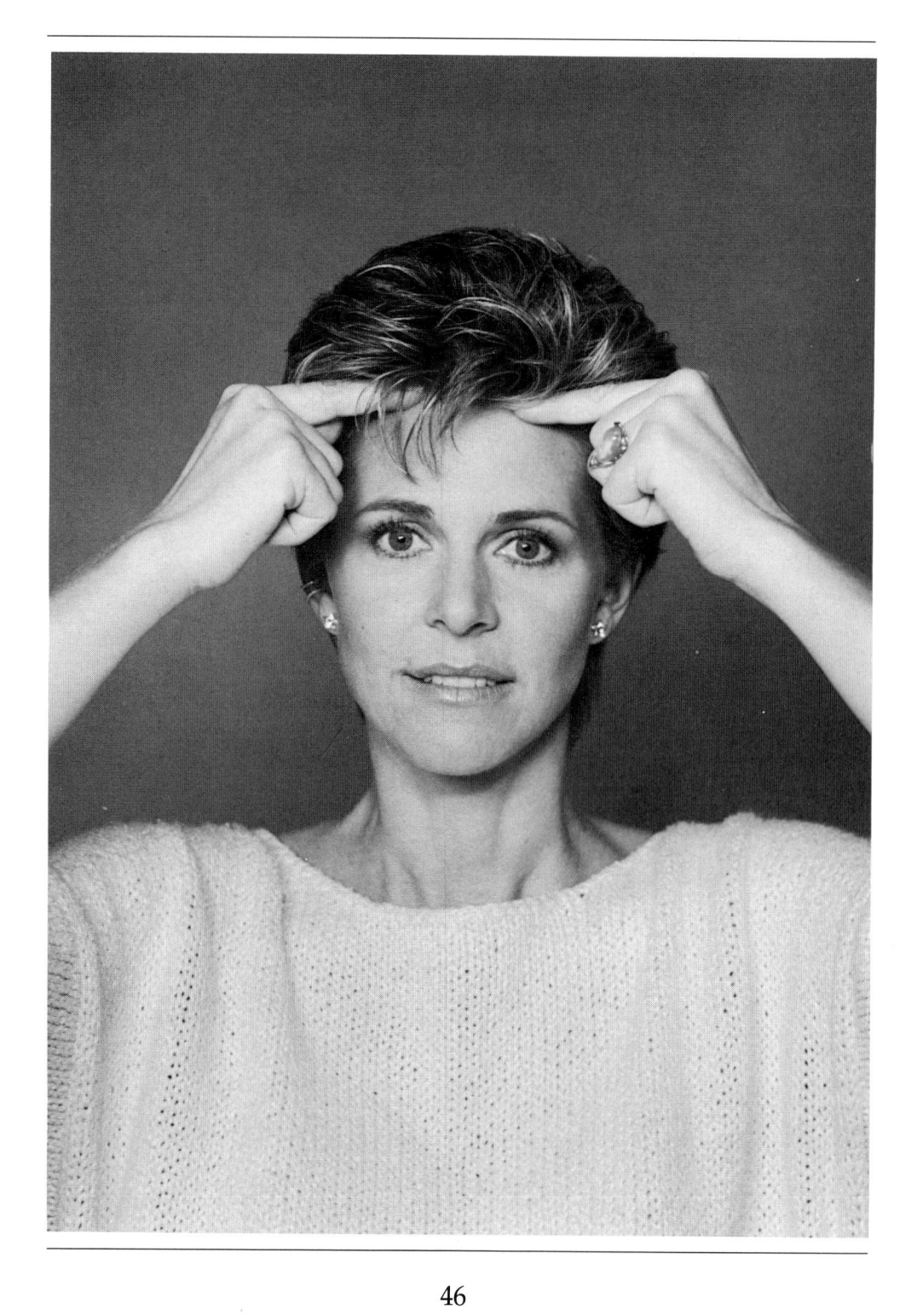

POINT 1

Located at your hairline, directly above your eyes.

Use firm pressure and make small inward circles.

This jump-off point for the program opens the flow of energy down into your face. The thin muscles in this area of the scalp and forehead will be relaxed and invigorated by the action of the massage.

This point is known in classical Oriental texts as *Mei Jung*. The massaging of it may cause you to experience some pleasant feelings in your abdomen, since this point sits astride a meridian line related to the gall bladder and liver. The point is one traditionally used to treat simple headaches.

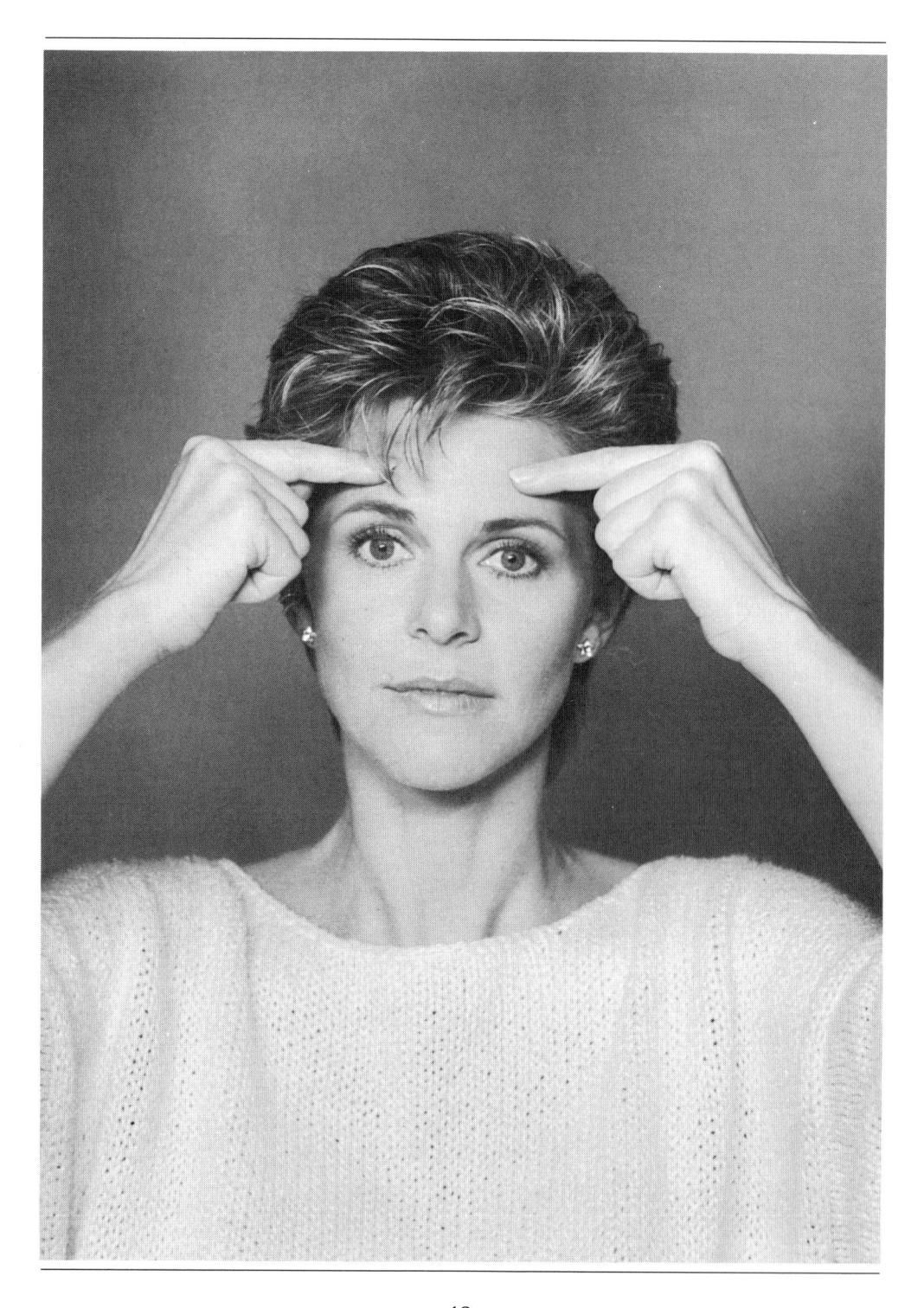

POINT 2

Located just below the previous point, midway between the hairline and the top of the eyebrow.

Again, make small, firm inward circles.

Massaging this point is very relaxing. You may feel some soothing warmth to the face and the back of the neck. Here you are working on the skin and muscles of the forehead. The muscles here support the layers of skin that, as years go by, have a tendency to develop deep wrinkles. By stimulating this point you will be building up that muscle tissue.

The point is called *Yang Bai*. It has been classically used for treating migraine headaches and insomnia.

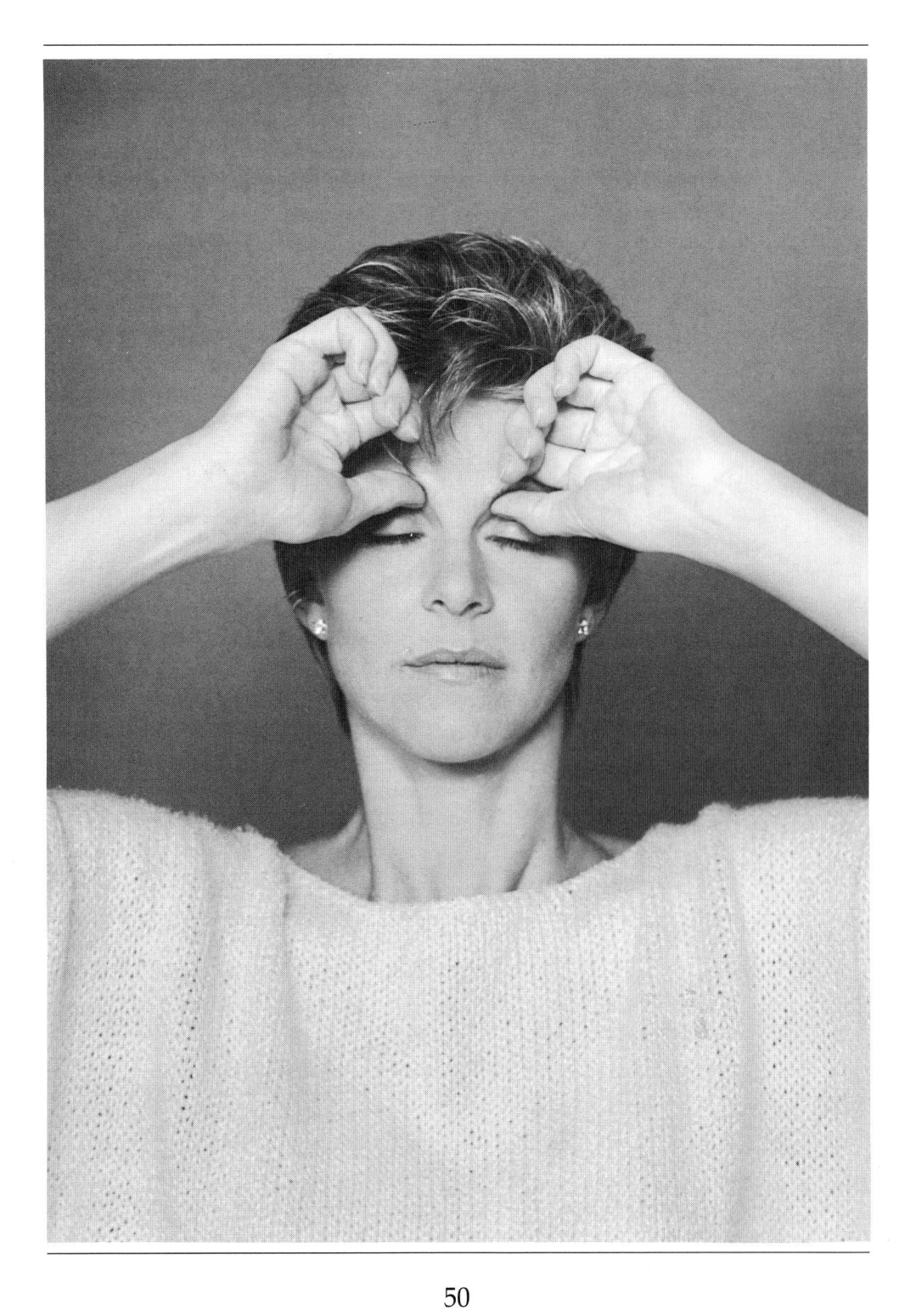

POINT 3

Located on the inside of your eye sockets next to your nose. On this point you will use your thumbs instead of your fingertips. Lodge your thumbs against each side of the base of the bridge of your nose; then rotate them upward, so that you push up and onto the bone and are right under the eyebrow. The thumb fits perfectly into the contour of the inside corner of the eyes here.

Make small inward circles, being careful not to push against your eyes.

Activation of this point stimulates the flow of energy down around the eyes, the nose, and into the center of your face.

This point is called *Zan Zhu*. It has been traditionally used for headache, eyestrain, and for discomfort around the eyes. It may also have an effect on the sinuses.

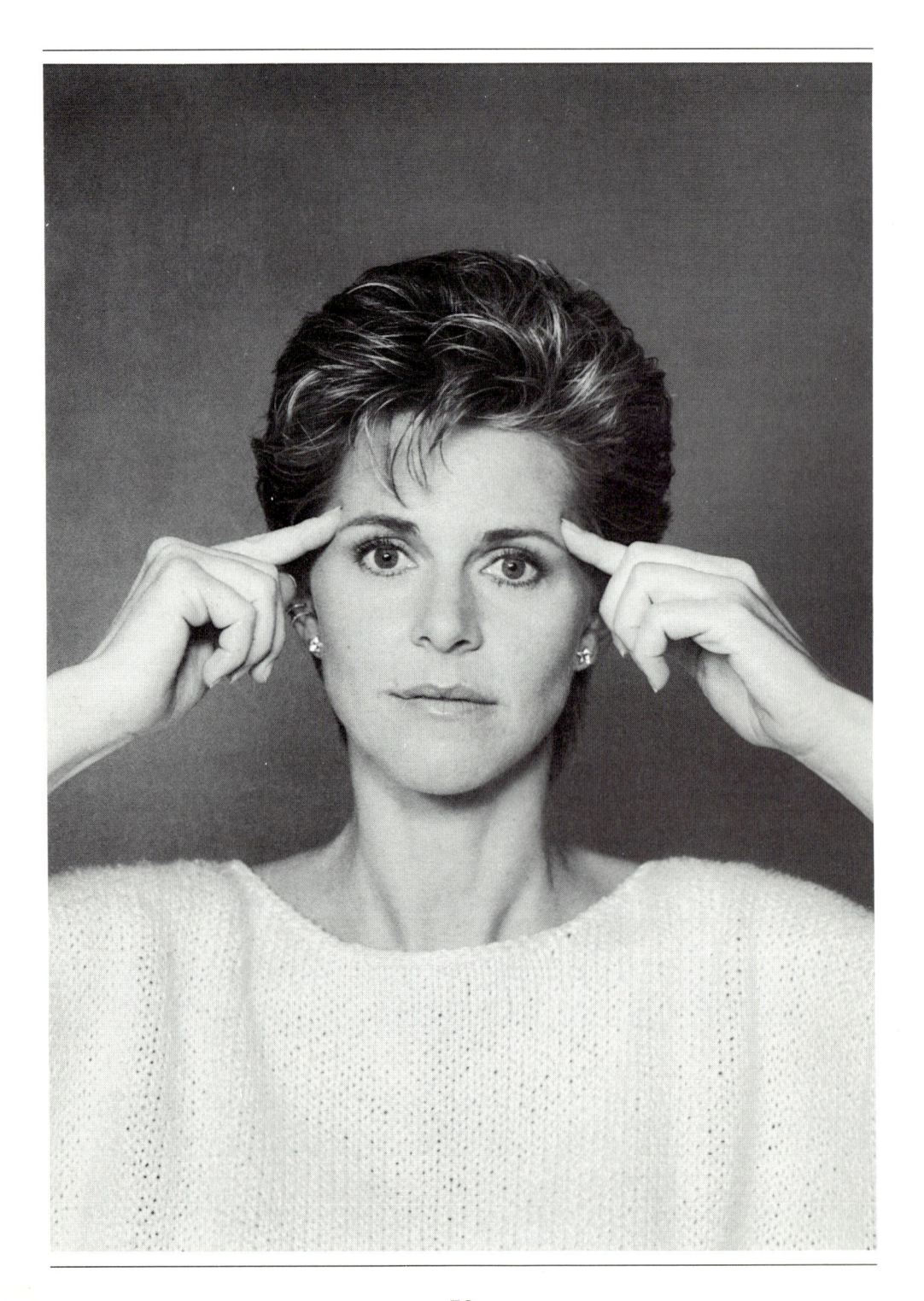

POINT 4

Located at the far ends of your eyebrows. This time make small outward circles.

At this point, you are working on the delicate muscle structure that is above the eye and the temples. It is helping to stimulate the muscles and bring them back to life. This is one of the points that is beneficial for crow's-feet, because it helps to fill out the tissue under which the creases develop.

Remember to try to keep your breathing rhythm. If you are aware of any tension in your shoulders, let them drop and relax. You may want to close your eyes while you massage this point.

The name of this point is *Sizhu Kong*. It, too, is known as an important point for the treatment of headaches.

After doing this massage, pause for a few seconds. Take a deep breath and vigorously shake out your hands.

54

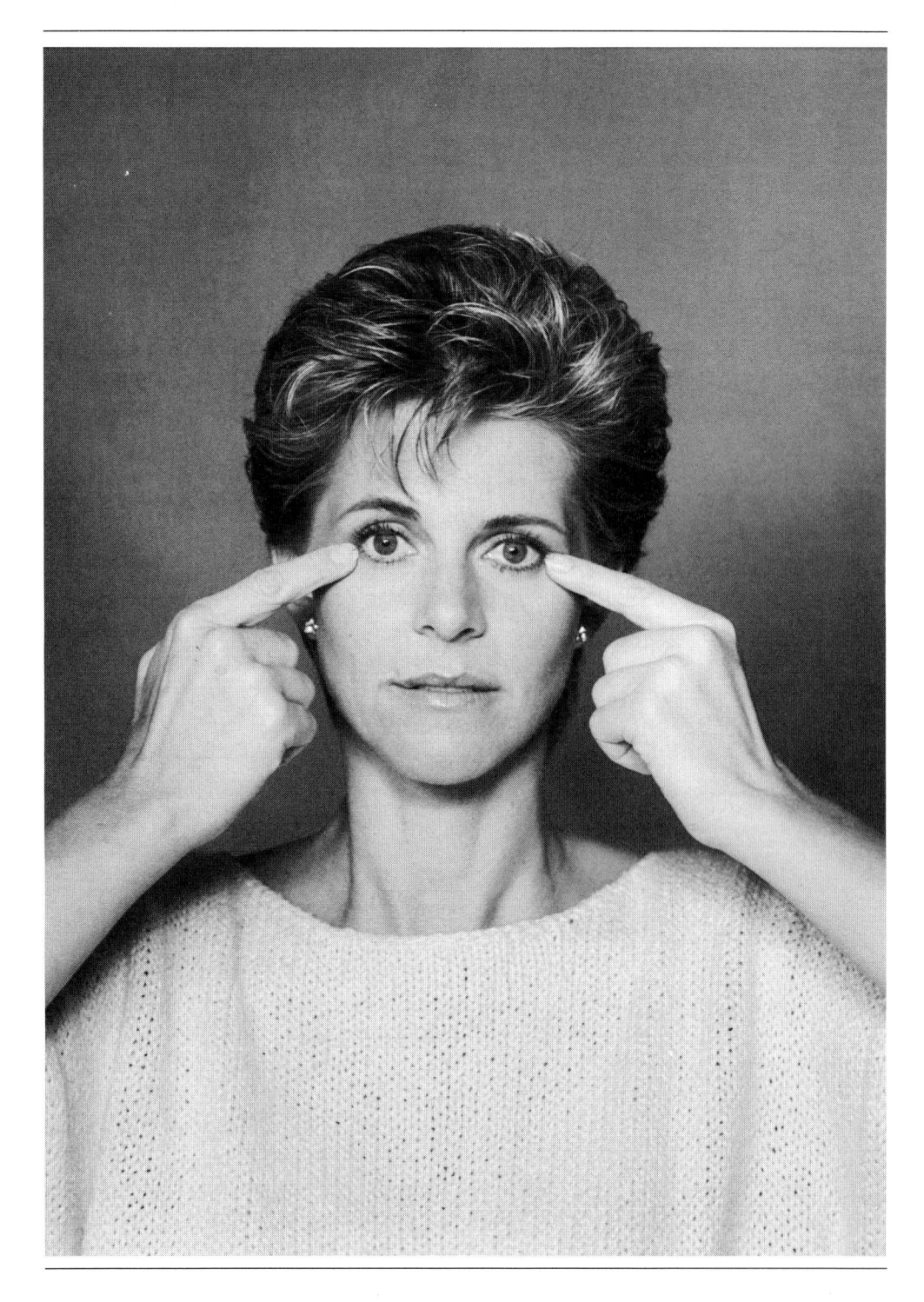

POINT 5

Located at the outside corner of your eyes. This is the area where crow's-feet begin to emerge.

Again, make small outward circles. Take care not to push against the eye. Feel for the little depression in the muscle and use firm pressure.

Here, too, you may want to close your eyes during the massage, and that's fine.

Massaging this point enhances circulation and energy to the eyes and the area of the eye sockets. The small muscles become invigorated and toned. The skin becomes supple and soft.

This point is called *Wai Ming*. It has been found helpful in treating irritated or dry eyes.

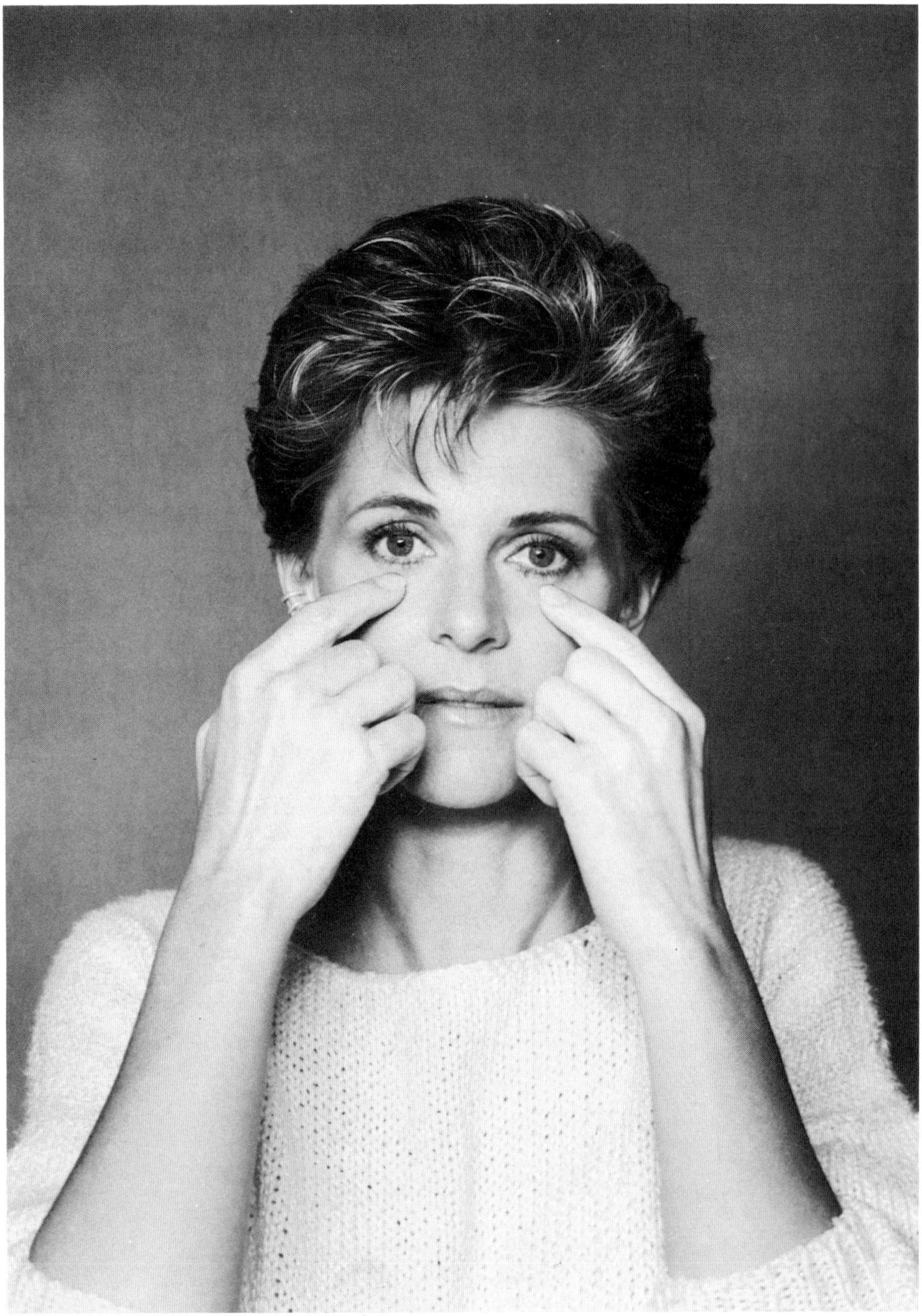

POINT 6

Located on the ridge of your eye sockets on a straight line down from your pupil. Feel for that ever so slight depression on the top of the cheekbone. There. That's the place.

Make small outward circles, being careful not to press on the eyes. The massage should be done right there on the ridge of the bone, in the area where unsightly "bags" develop. Stimulation of this point helps restore tone to local muscle tissue, resulting usually in a pleasing improvement of the condition and appearance of the skin below the eyes.

This point is called *Cheng Qi*, and it is known to have a beneficial effect on eyestrain and tension around the eyes.

58

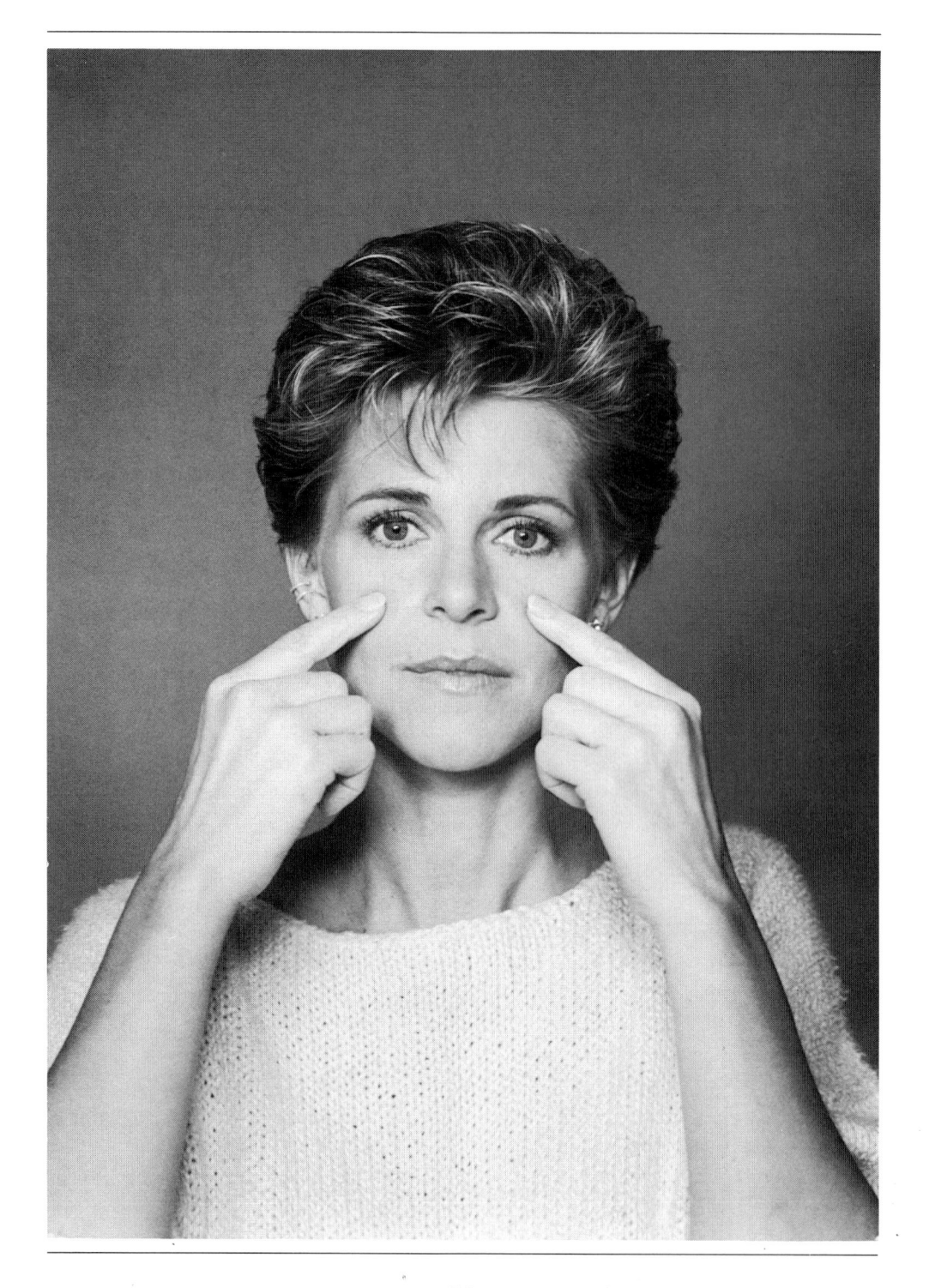

POINT 7

Continuing straight down from the pupil again, you will pass Point 6 to a line about even with the flare of your nostrils. You will find a depression there in your cheek, and that's where the point is.

Make small outward circles.

Massaging this point works on the large muscle in the cheek, helping to fill out sunken tissue and restore the natural angles of your face. Circulation is also enhanced, bringing with it the healthy glow of rosy cheeks that we all admire.

This point is called *Sibai*. It is known to have beneficial effects on the sinuses.

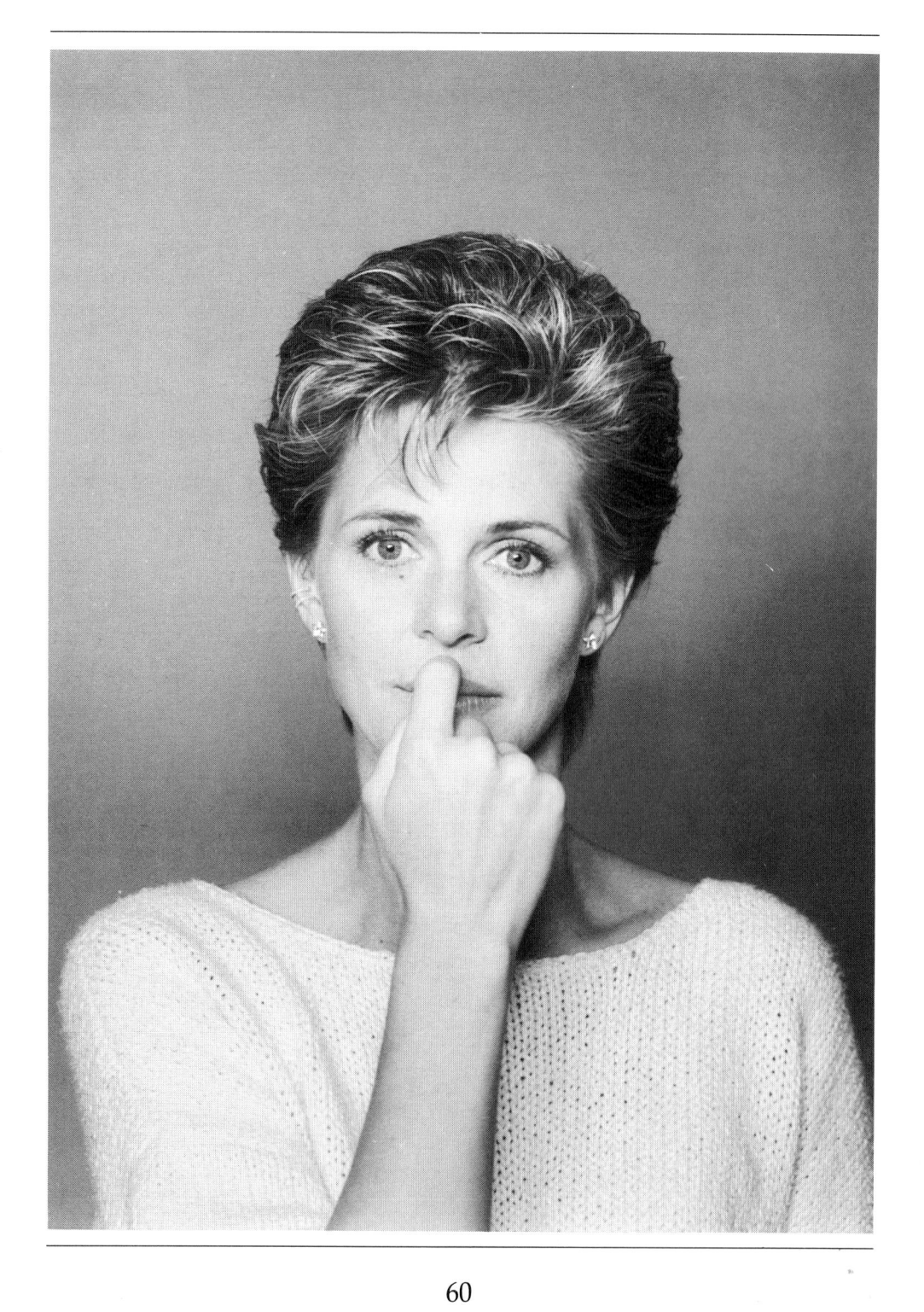

POINT 8

Located in your naso-labial cleft, midway between the bottom of your nose and the top of your lip.

Make small clockwise circles with firm pressure.

Stimulating this area is helpful for the vertical lines that appear below the nose and the upper lip.

This point is called *Ren Zhong*. It is well known in acupuncture as an "emergency" point for fainting, dizziness, and nausea.

You have had your hands up for a while now and they may be getting tired. Perhaps there is some tension building in the shoulders. So take a momentary pause. Let your hands fall on your lap. Take a deep breath and now shake out your hands again.

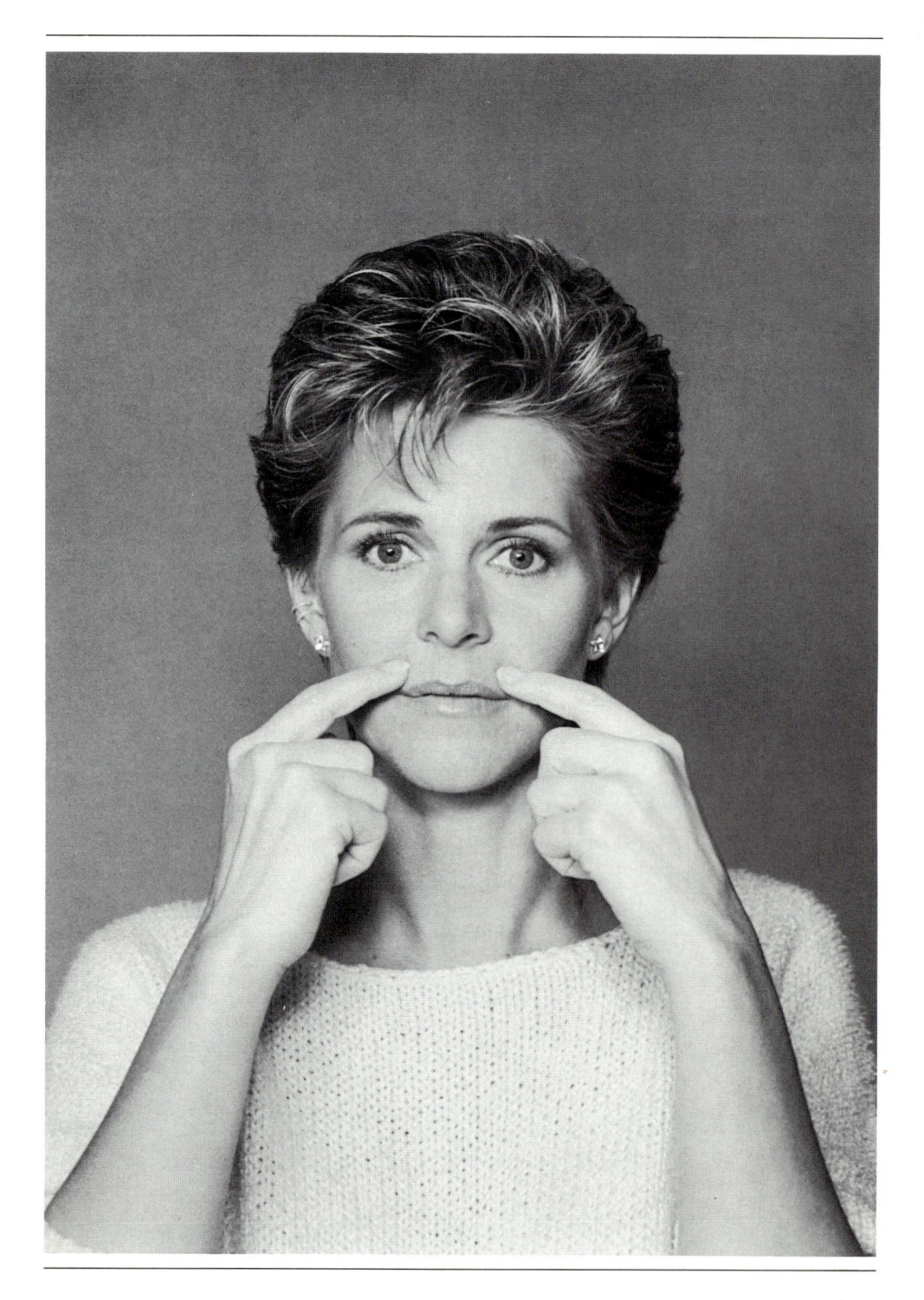

POINT 9

Located above your upper lip about half an inch from the outside corners of your mouth.

Make small outward circles with firm pressure.

This point has a positive effect on the small wrinkles around the corners of the mouth.

The point is called *Dicang*.

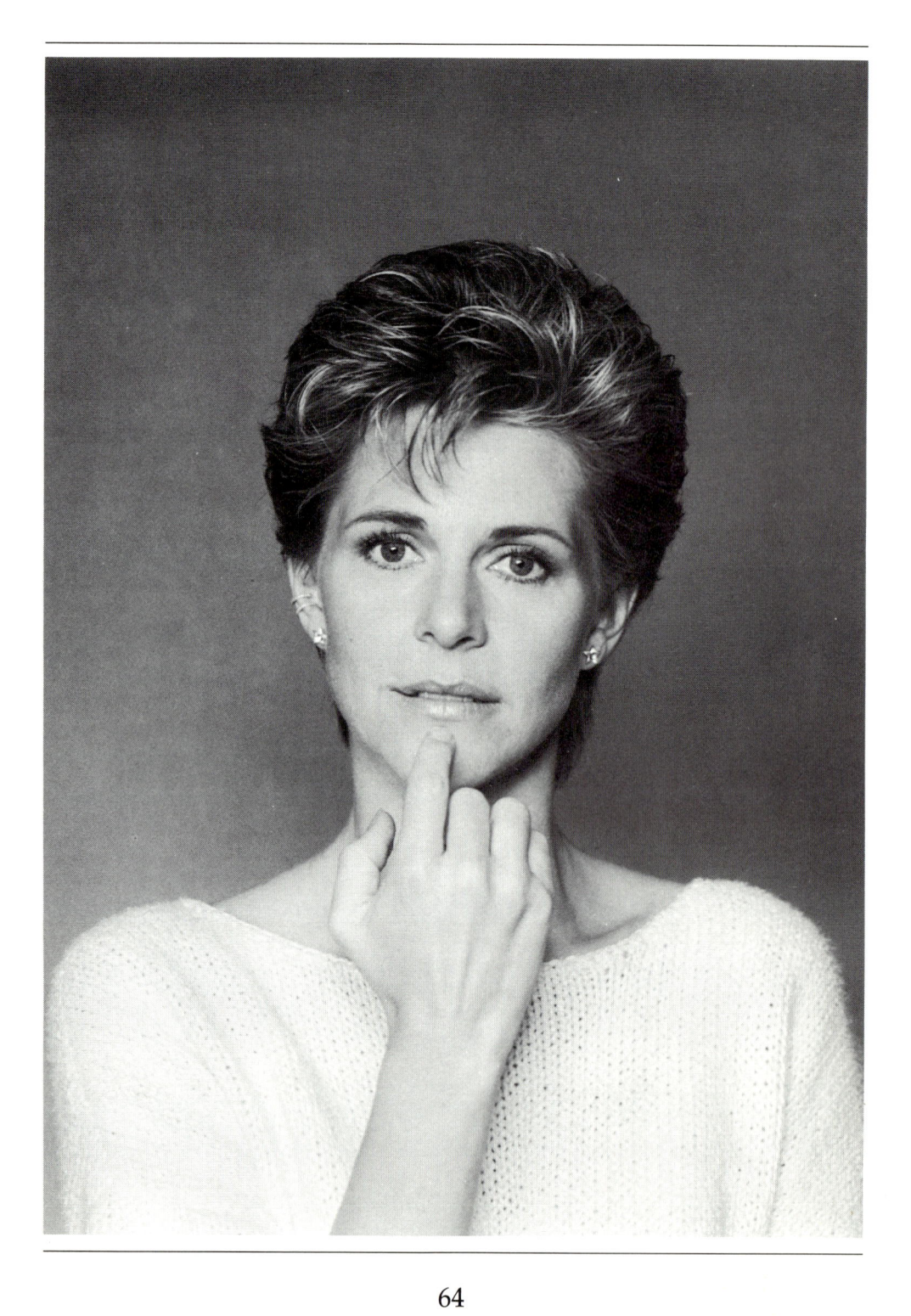

POINT 10

Located midway between your lower lip and your chin. Make small clockwise circles.

This action helps to lessen the little wrinkles on the chin. This is a gateway point that channels circulation and energy up to the area of the mouth and face beyond. Massage here has a relaxing effect on tension in the lower jaw.

The point is called *Cheng Jiang*.

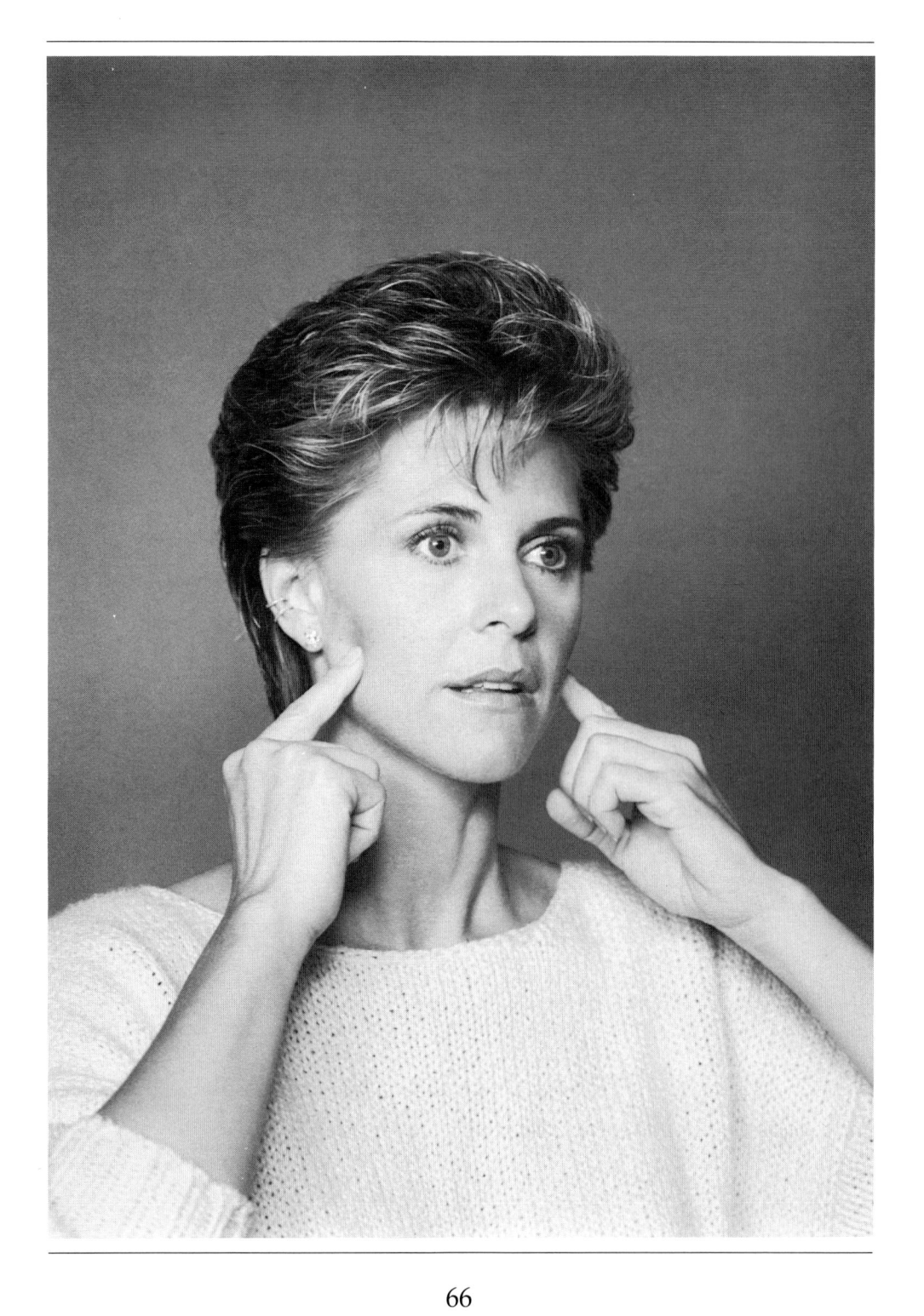

POINT 11

Located on the big muscle at the hinge of the jaw. Let your mouth fall slightly open. Your fingers will find a depression in the muscle where the point is situated.

Make small circles, starting toward the back of your head.

This point is useful for dealing with tension in the jaw and enhances the flow of energy into the entire face.

The point is called *Chia Che*.

LINDSAY: *I know that I carry facial tension in this place, so often I will work this spot during any particularly stressful situation. I find it usually helps to eliminate the tension in quick order.*

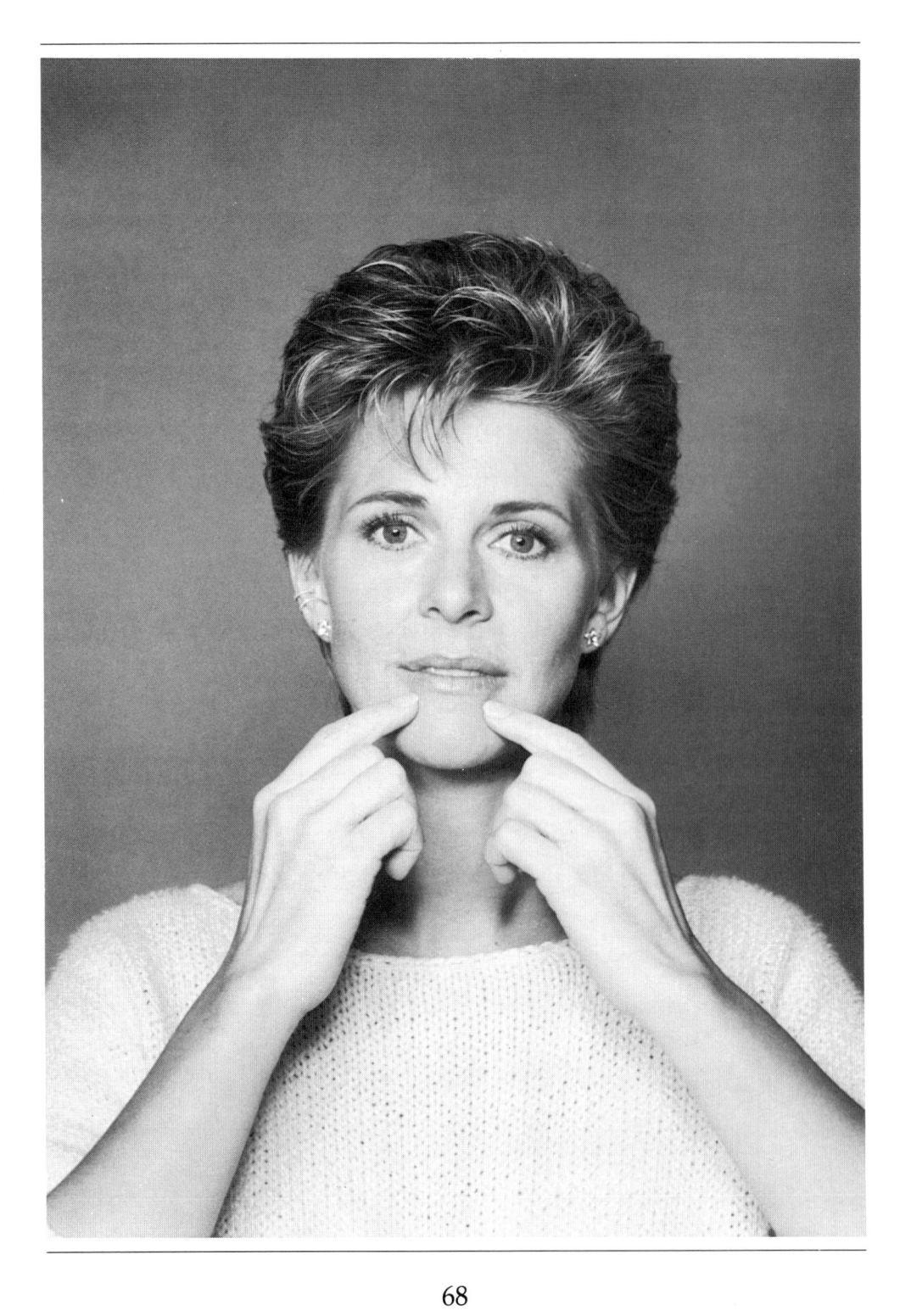

POINT 12

Located midway between your chin and lower lip, approximately half an inch from the corner of your mouth.

Make small outward circles.

This point is helpful for those lines around the corners of the mouth and for toning the muscles of the chin. Remember, you can use either your fingertips (as shown here) or your knuckles throughout the Acupressure Facelift.

This particular spot on the face does not have a name in classical acupuncture texts.

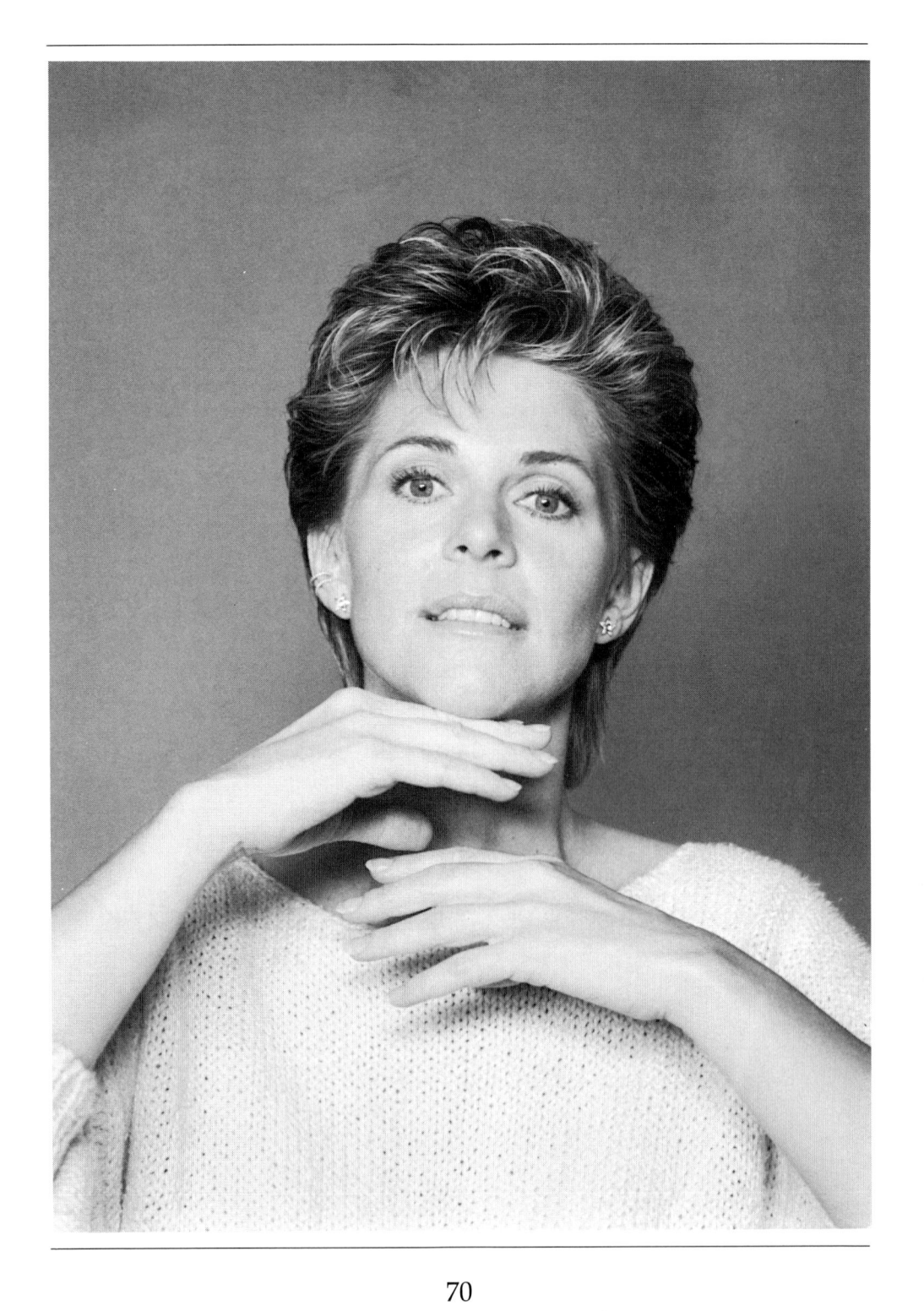

CHIN SLAP

Now do some quick rhythmic slapping on the skin and tissue that often tend to sag just below your chin. Stick your chin out and use the backs of both hands alternately to beat out a stimulating massage against the flesh.

There is no need to slap hard, just firmly enough to feel the circulation being stimulated. The slapping action helps to firm up sagging muscle tissue.

Do this exercise for about thirty seconds.

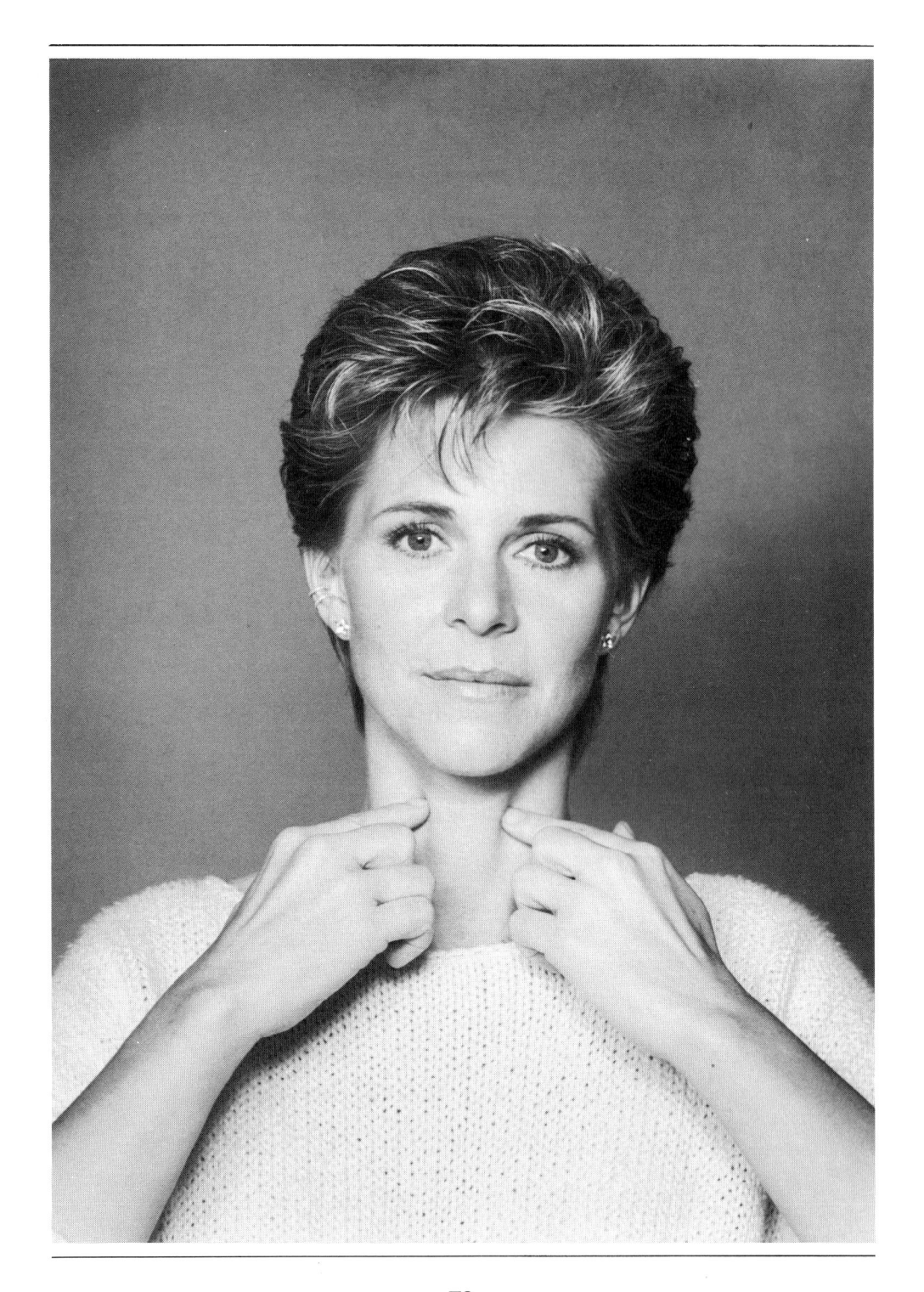

POINT 13

Bring your fingers to your throat midway on your neck at both sides of the windpipe. You may have to lean your head back a little to get at these spots.

This massage uses a vibrating motion—quickly up and down. Use firm pressure, but do not push hard enough to restrict the flow of your breathing.

This point stimulates the area of the thyroid gland and tends to generate energy throughout the body. It helps to tone up local muscle and flabby tissue found on the mid neck and throat.

The point is called *Ren Ying*.

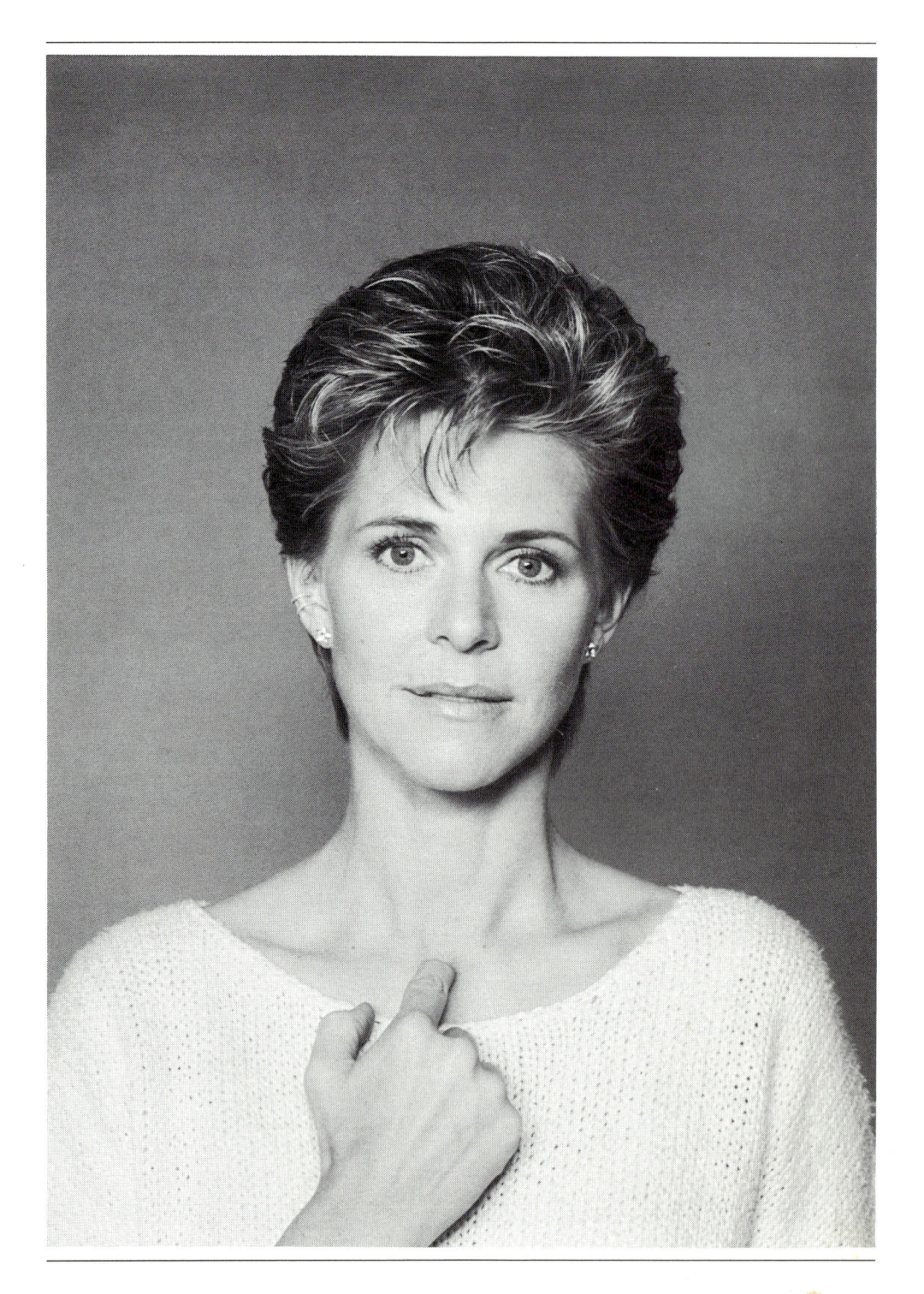

POINT 14

Located in the notch of the bone at the base of your throat.

Stay on the bone and make small circles. Be careful not to push into your windpipe.

This point opens up important pathways of energy into the neck and head from the body.

The point is called *Tian Tu*. It is an important point used in treating coughs and hoarseness.

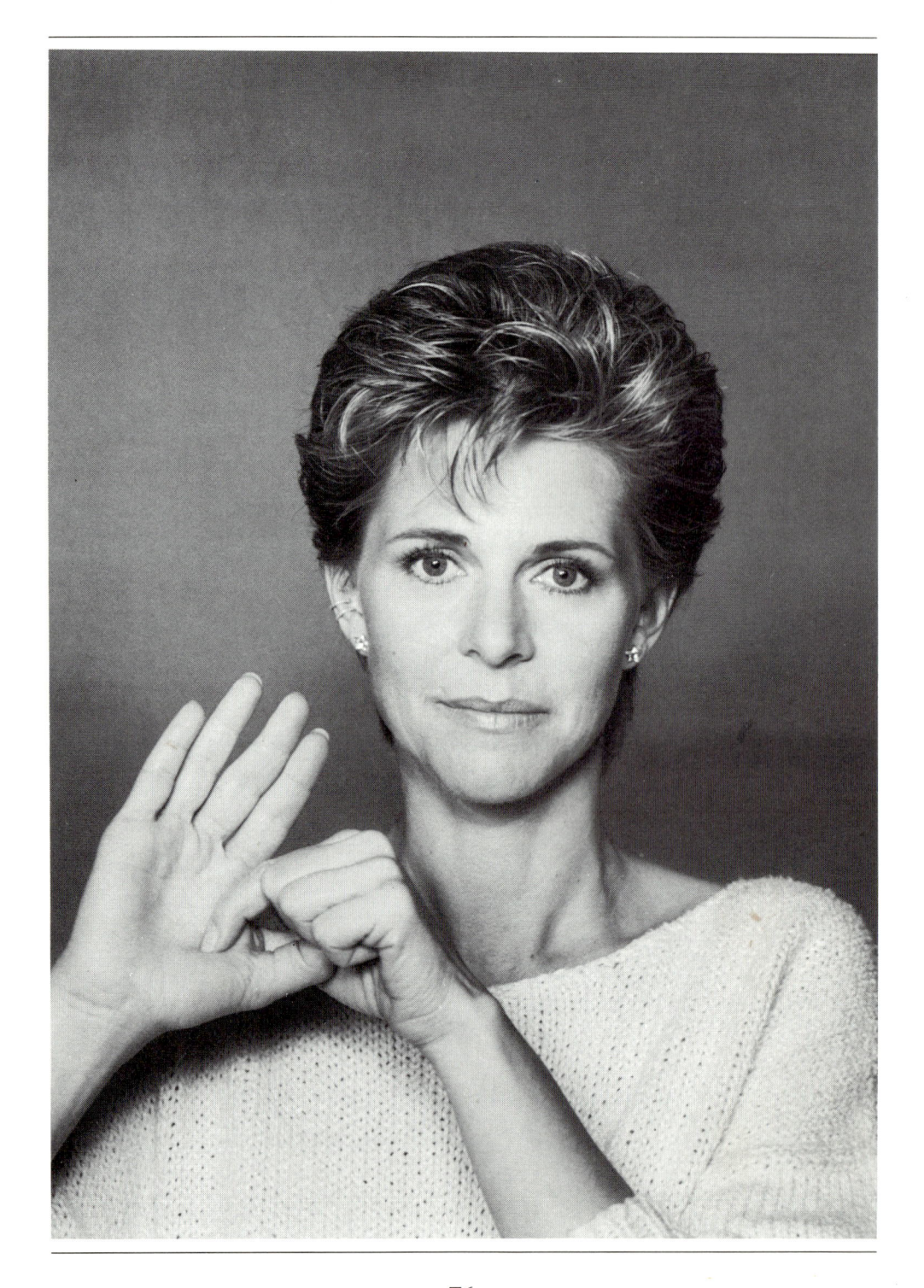

POINT 15

Located on each of your hands in the soft "webbed" tissue where the thumb and forefinger come together.

Using the tip of your thumb and forefinger of your left hand, feel for the point on your right hand. Massage deep into this space with a circular motion for one minute.

This point is called *Ho Ku* and is one of the master points in the body for stimulating the flow of energy to the entire head and neck. This point is classically used for headache and tooth pain and has a beneficial effect on digestion.

Although this and the next three points are not located in the face and neck region, they are still important for our purposes because they correspond to and nurture many areas of the head.

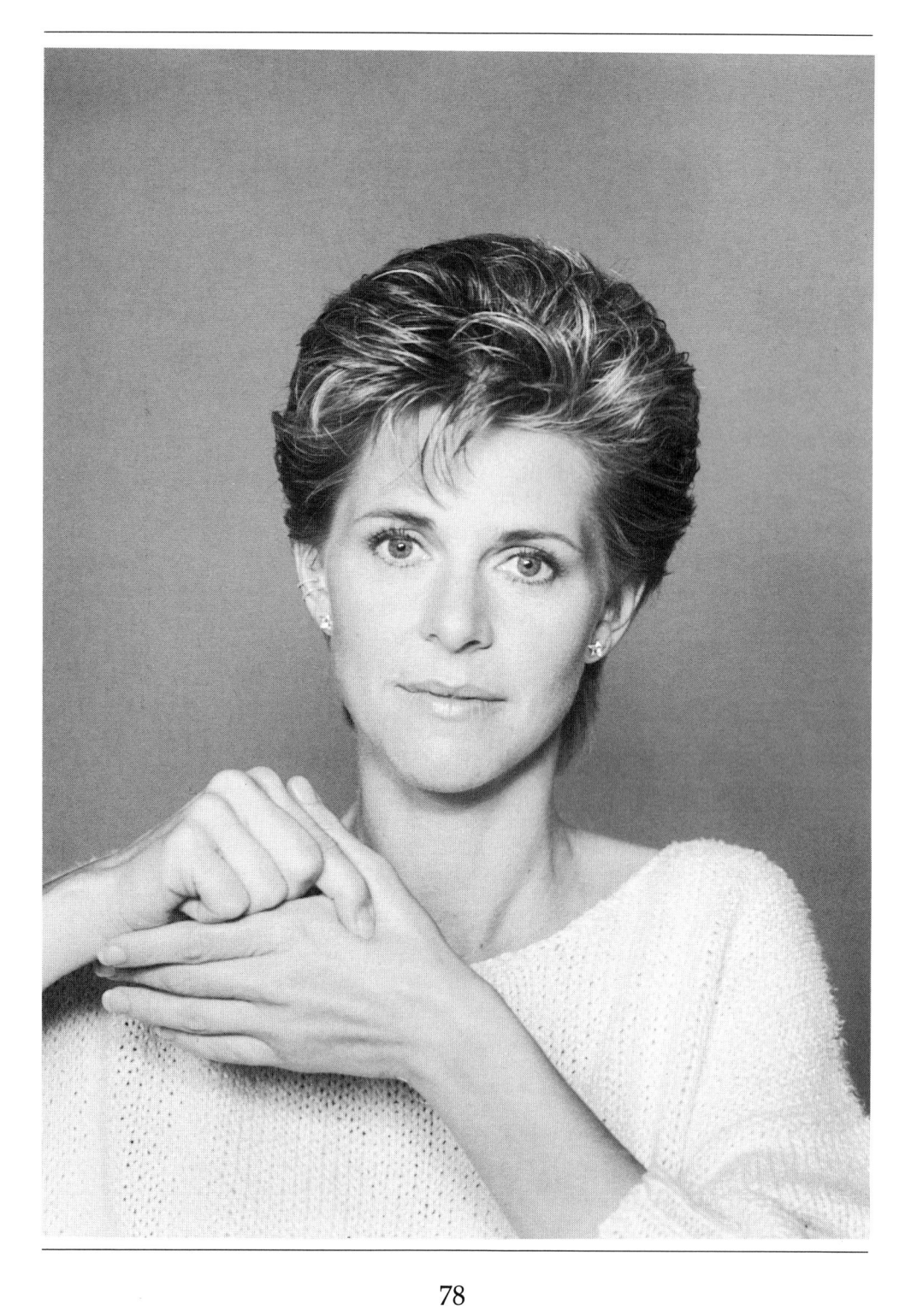

POINT 16

Now change to the other hand and proceed exactly as you did for Point 15.

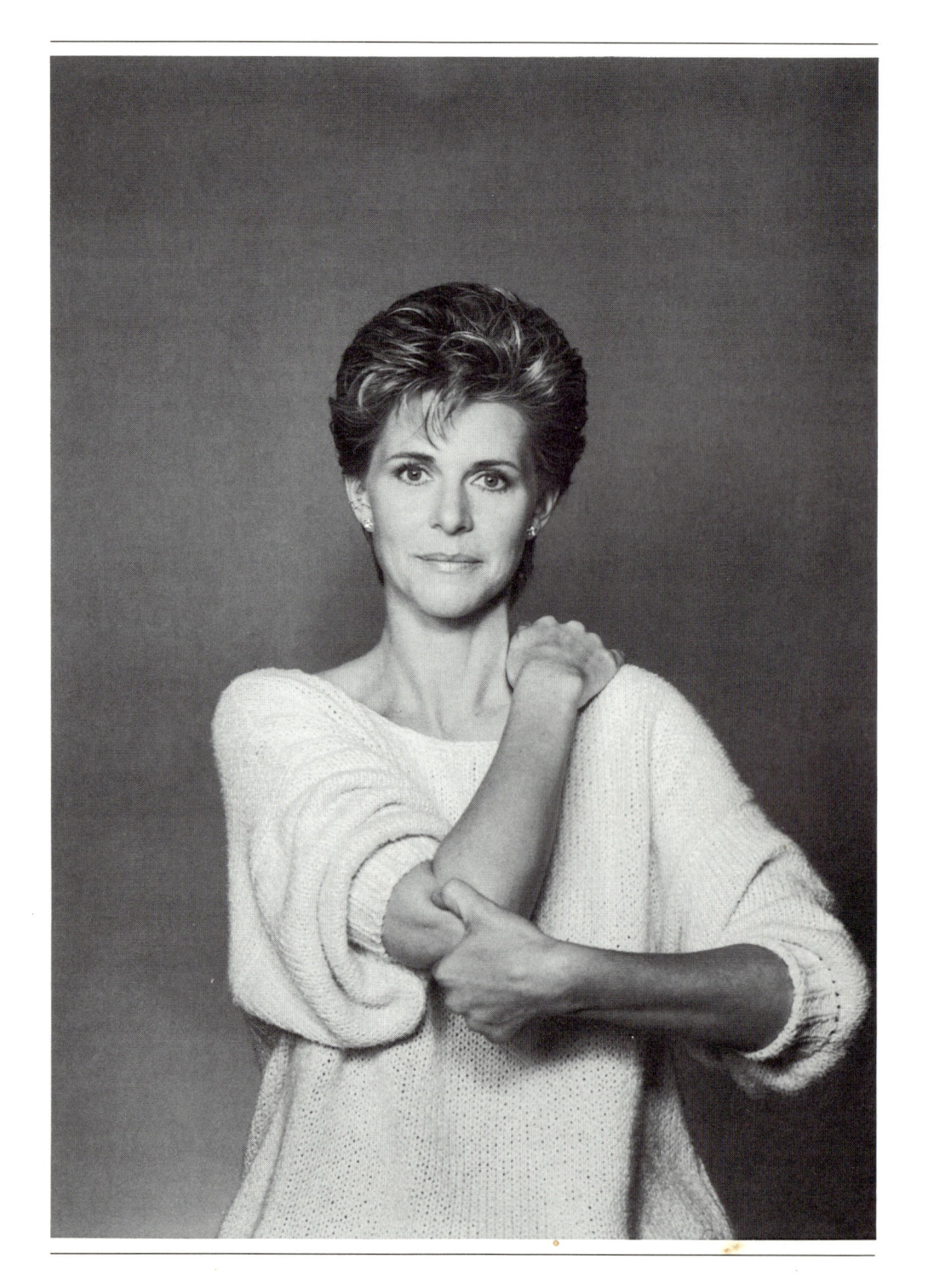

POINT 17

Located on the right arm at the base of the crease of the elbow. To find the point accurately, put your right hand on your left shoulder. Look down and follow the crease that is formed by bending the elbow. At the base of that crease, you will find a notchlike hole just above and against the bone. This is the point.

Push in with your left thumb and massage deep into this point. Use a circular motion. Again, this is feeding energy up to the face, head, and neck.

The name of this point is *Chu Chih*. It is used in acupuncture for the treatment of the skin in general.

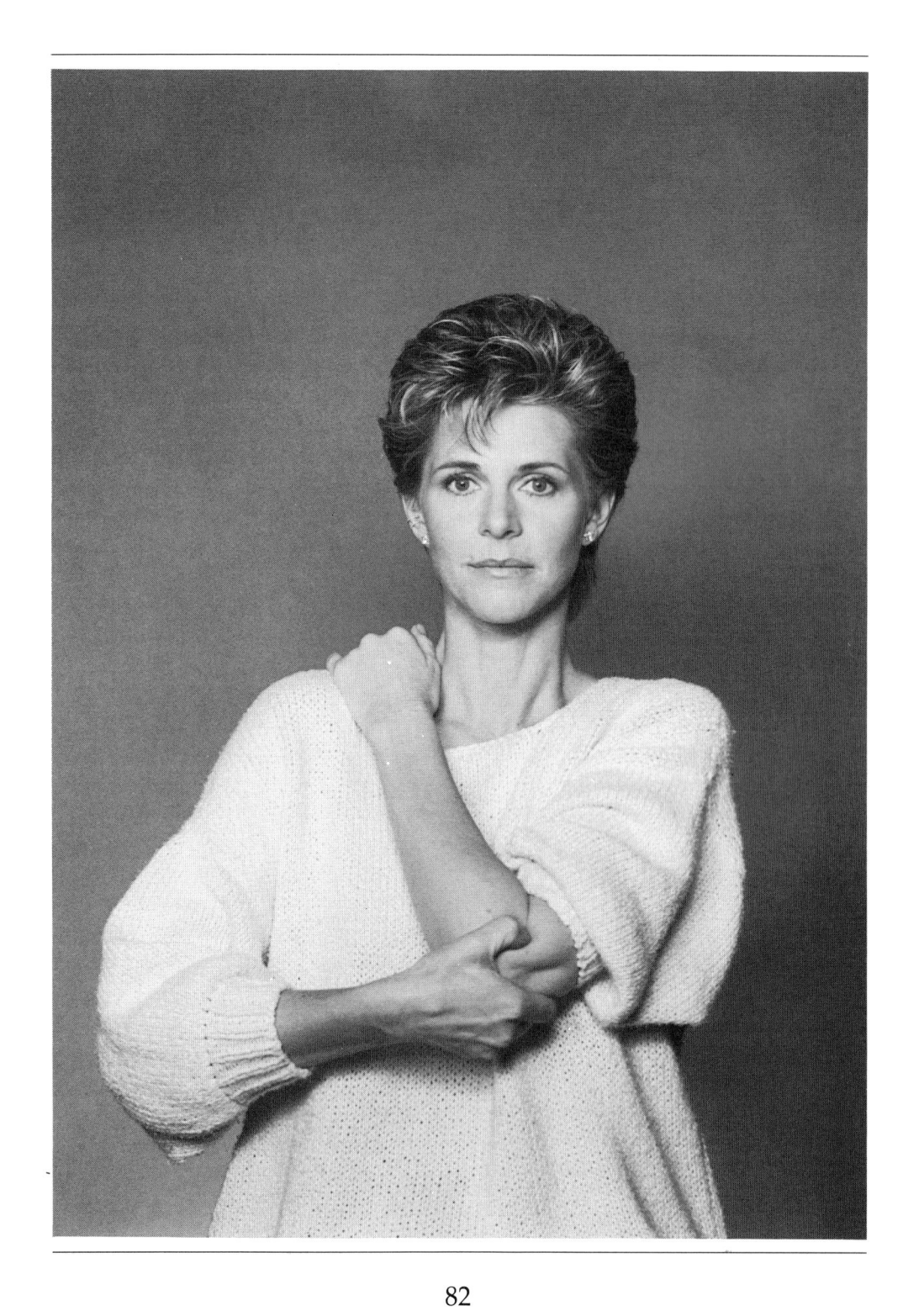

POINT 18

Now change to the other arm and proceed as you did for Point No. 17.

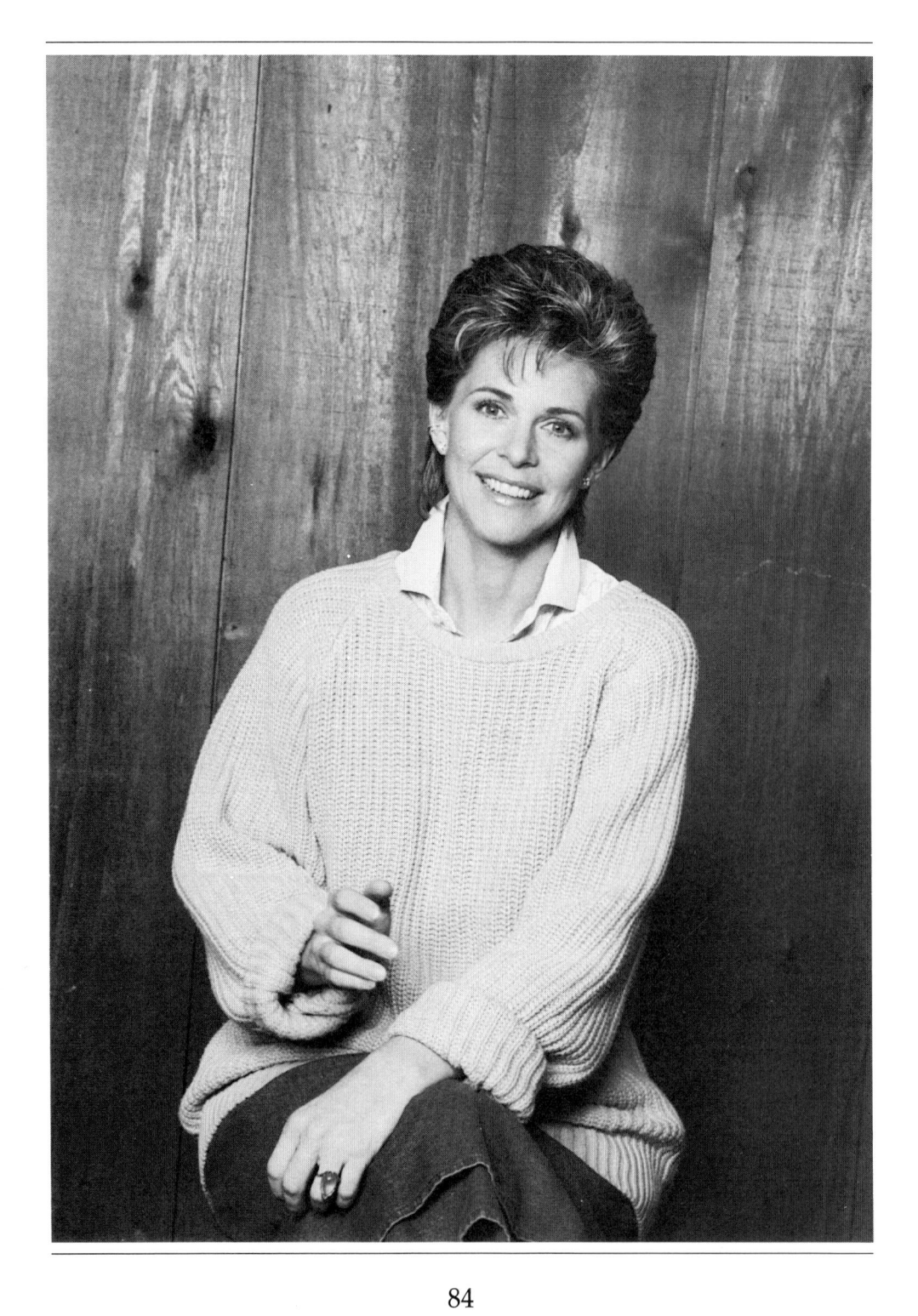

QUESTIONS AND ANSWERS

Whenever we are out talking to people about the Acupressure Facelift, the most common question we hear is this: "Does it really work?"

The answer is a short and simple "yes."

"Just try it yourself and experience the improvement," we say.

"Well, then, just how fast does it work?" they also want to know.

"You begin to both feel and see results immediately," we answer. "There is renewed circulation to the skin, bringing with it a natural, youthful glow and radiance. After a week or so, you will begin to see a lessening of wrinkles and facial lines. This process will turn the lights back on in your face."

LINDSAY: *I am often asked about how I can fit this program into a busy day. I answer that you just have to make a commitment to yourself. Here is something that is very beneficial for you; something you can do to help yourself. So you find the time, whether that means getting up twenty minutes earlier or going to bed twenty minutes later. I sometimes say to my kids, "Mom needs twenty minutes for herself and I'll be right back."*

Look at it another way: We have been taught to brush our teeth since we were little, and we find time to do that, no matter how busy our day is. We do it because it is something we have to do to keep our teeth and gums in good health. Similarly if you consider your face and appearance a priority matter, then you will set aside the time to do the massage.

We are asked a whole variety of questions, and we thought we would share the most commonly asked ones with you, along with the answers.

QUESTION: Does the Acupressure Facelift have permanent benefits?

ANSWER: Benefits are permanent so long as the massage is maintained. After you have done the massage regularly for thirty days, the skin and muscles of your face will improve to the point where you can maintain the gains with just a few sessions a week. The Acupressure Facelift is an exercise program. Your facial muscles will respond to exercise in the same way as the rest of your body. You cannot expect to exercise once, twice, or three times, or for a week, and have the results last forever.

QUESTION: Does everybody obtain maximum results by thirty days?

ANSWER: Progress is, of course, an individual matter. However, generally, it seems that completion of the rebuilding process occurs by thirty days. Some cases will take longer because of individual conditions, ailments, energy systems, or age.

Use this as a guideline: When you feel you have reached the

point where you have achieved the results you want, then drop down to the maintenance schedule. This could be well beyond the thirty days in some cases.

Quite a few people we know try to keep up the daily program even after they have obtained the desired cosmetic results because of the relaxation benefit they receive.

QUESTION: If I stop the program, will my face return to its previous condition?

ANSWER: That depends. If you stop altogether, the chances are that, after a period of time, your face will return to its previous appearance. By adhering to the maintenance program of a few massages a week, you can keep up your healthy glow. You have to do it to get it . . . and keep it.

Once you are into the program, however, and you stop for a few weeks or so, you will not really lose any noticeable ground. Just get back into it as soon as you can.

QUESTION: Do I have to follow the massage points in order?

ANSWER: It is important to follow the order as we have outlined it in the preceding chapter. You should start at the top and work down. That follows the natural flow of energy in your body.

If you skip points or do them in a random order, there is no harm done; nor does it mean that the massage will be ineffective. However, experience has shown that best results are obtained by following the order sequentially as we have presented it.

QUESTION: Does the massage eliminate aging spots and sun spots?

ANSWER: No. It may, however, render them less apparent, as you restore more circulation to the skin.

There was one dramatic case of a woman whose face was full of premature wrinkles and aging spots (similar to what we call "liver spots"). She looked much older than her years, perhaps due to stress caused by her very high-pressure job. At any rate, she started the massages and concurrently changed other things in her life—eating better and starting an exercise program. She began to feel better and look better, as a result of making these changes. Her tired, pale skin began to radiate with a glow of health. In time the spots seemed to fade, becoming considerably less noticeable, and the wrinkles softened to a considerable degree.

QUESTION: Can it help seventy-five-year-old (or older) skin that is heavily wrinkled?

ANSWER: Yes, it will make a difference. Facial muscles are facial muscles, no matter what the age. However, in traditional Oriental medicine it is known that, the longer you have a condition, the longer it usually takes to treat and restore normalcy. You may have to work a little harder and longer, but the results will be well worth it.

The massage will not make you look eighteen, but your face will look better and feel better.

QUESTION: Will the massage eliminate acne scars?

ANSWER: No. Unfortunately, scarring is a permanent condition.

However, by invigorating the circulation and revitalizing the muscles, the skin becomes more healthy, takes on a natural color, and fills out. These changes tend to render the scars less noticeable.

QUESTION: Is it possible that I will look fat because the facial muscles are filling out?

ANSWER: No. The massage will bring the skin and the underlying muscle layer to a normal state. Your skin will never puff out abnormally or appear to be swollen.

QUESTION: Are the pressure points easy to find?

ANSWER: After a while, you learn precisely where all of them are and it will become second nature. With practice your fingers will go right to them.

At the very beginning, you will probably poke around and search for the locations. That's why we have illustrated the points for you. Use the pictures as a guide until you learn the territory.

QUESTION: Does the Acupressure Facelift work for men, too?

ANSWER: Whiskered, bearded, or clean-shaven, a man's face reacts the same way. You get a natural muscle tone, softening of wrinkles, and a healthful glow, which all add up to looking better and younger. The pressure points for men are in exactly the same places as for women.

QUESTION: If I have a sunburned face should I do the massage?

ANSWER: It is preferable that you don't. The skin will be painful, tender, and maybe even swollen. Wait until the irritation subsides.

Excess sun is very damaging to the skin. The potential for skin cancer is well publicized. Instead of baking your face and taking chances, why not use the Acupressure Massage to supply it with a natural color and glow? When you are out in the sun, apply a sunscreen or wear a hat. Your skin will thank you in the years ahead.

QUESTION: Are there any other particular conditions or times when I shouldn't do the technique?

ANSWER: If you have a blemish or cut, or if you have injured yourself, don't massage that particular area. Wait until the condition heals.

If you have had surgery on your face, wait until the area heals. Never do anything that could disturb the healing process.

QUESTION: Can I watch TV while doing the massage?

ANSWER: Once you are well familiar with the pressure points and don't need to concentrate on finding them, you can watch TV while you do it. However, it is unlikely that you will get any relaxation benefits from the technique if you are watching the news or a horror film while doing it.

> LINDSAY: *To get the maximum benefits, whenever you do the entire program you really want to put your attention on yourself and not be distracted. A lot of people like to listen to music when they do it. Classical, soft jazz, or any relaxing music, whatever you like best. Some people even do the procedure to the rhythm of the music. That works fine, too.*

QUESTION: Can I do it while talking on the phone?

ANSWER: Sure. Lots of people do. Simply hold the phone with one hand and massage one side of your face with your free hand. Then switch hands and repeat the procedure on the other side of your face.

QUESTION: Can I start the Acupressure Facelift before I start to develop wrinkles and sagging skin?

ANSWER: Yes, and it is a good idea to do so. If you believe in exercise for the health of your body, then you should also regard this massage as a form of facial fitness. Why not do for your face what you do for your whole body? The same principle applies.

Think of it as good prevention. By regularly massaging your face, you keep the circulation and energy channels clear and flowing with the kind of nutrition necessary for healthy skin. You keep the skin and muscles supple. You can retard the appearance of wrinkles and spots and maintain a youthful glow longer in life.

The ancient Chinese placed great stock in the preventive and youth-sustaining effect of this procedure.

QUESTION: If you start again after stopping for a few weeks or even months, should you begin with the once-a-day program for a month or the maintenance program of two or three times weekly?

ANSWER: Do it once a day for thirty days or until you achieve the results you want. Since you have already done the procedure, your facial muscles are going to harbor "memory" of their previous improvement. Depending on how long you have been off the program, it probably should not take quite as long as it did initially to regain condition.

QUESTION: Will this technique help me if I have already had facial surgery?

ANSWER: Yes, but it may take longer than if there had not been an operation. Surgery cuts and damages the delicate meridian lines of energy that flow through and around the face. Moreover, scar tissue left in the wake of incisions tends to block or slow down the flow of energy.

QUESTION: I don't always have the fifteen or twenty minutes to do the procedure. Is there a miniversion of the Acupressure Facelift?

ANSWER: The program works best and you get maximum benefits if you do it the way we recommend. If you don't have the time to get it all in, then just focus on the areas of the face that concern you the most. If it is "bags" under your eyes or crow's-feet, then just do the points for those. You will get results, but not as many as if you were to do the whole program.

QUESTION: Can I concentrate on localized areas of wrinkles, or other areas that are of concern to me?

ANSWER: If you have specific areas of problems, you can put in some extra time on those spots. However, for maximum overall results, be sure to complete the entire massage first.

QUESTION: What causes "bags" under the eyes and does this program work to eliminate them?

ANSWER: What happens is that the muscles below the eyes often weaken and break down, permitting fat particles to herniate through them and push outward. You then see the "bags" or pouches commonly associated with aging or dissipation.

As you massage these places, the muscles around the eyes regain tone and firmness and become more effective in holding back the fat. Many women with a particularly serious condition have reported significant improvement. We cannot talk about "curing" anything, but we do say it will probably stop the process and improve appearances.

QUESTION: Should I do the massage in front of a mirror?

ANSWER: It is a good idea in the beginning until you become familiar with the procedure. Sitting in front of a mirror will help you find the points. You can also check what you are doing with the pictures in this book.

QUESTION: What is an Acupuncture Facelift?

ANSWER: Some acupuncturists perform facelifts involving a series of treatments using acupuncture needles. The procedure stimulates energy to the face and revitalizes muscle and skin, just as the Acupressure Facelift does without needles. We feel that the Acupressure Facelift gives you the satisfying opportunity to improve your health and beauty. It is a lifetime tool that brings welcome gifts of well-being every time you use it.

If you still have questions or comments after reading the instructions and the question-and-answer section, then feel free to write us. Send a self-addressed stamped envelope to: New Beauty, c/o Johnson/Klein, 12413 Ventura Court, Suite D, Studio City, CA 91604.

PART III
LINDSAY WAGNER'S TOTAL APPROACH TO BEAUTY

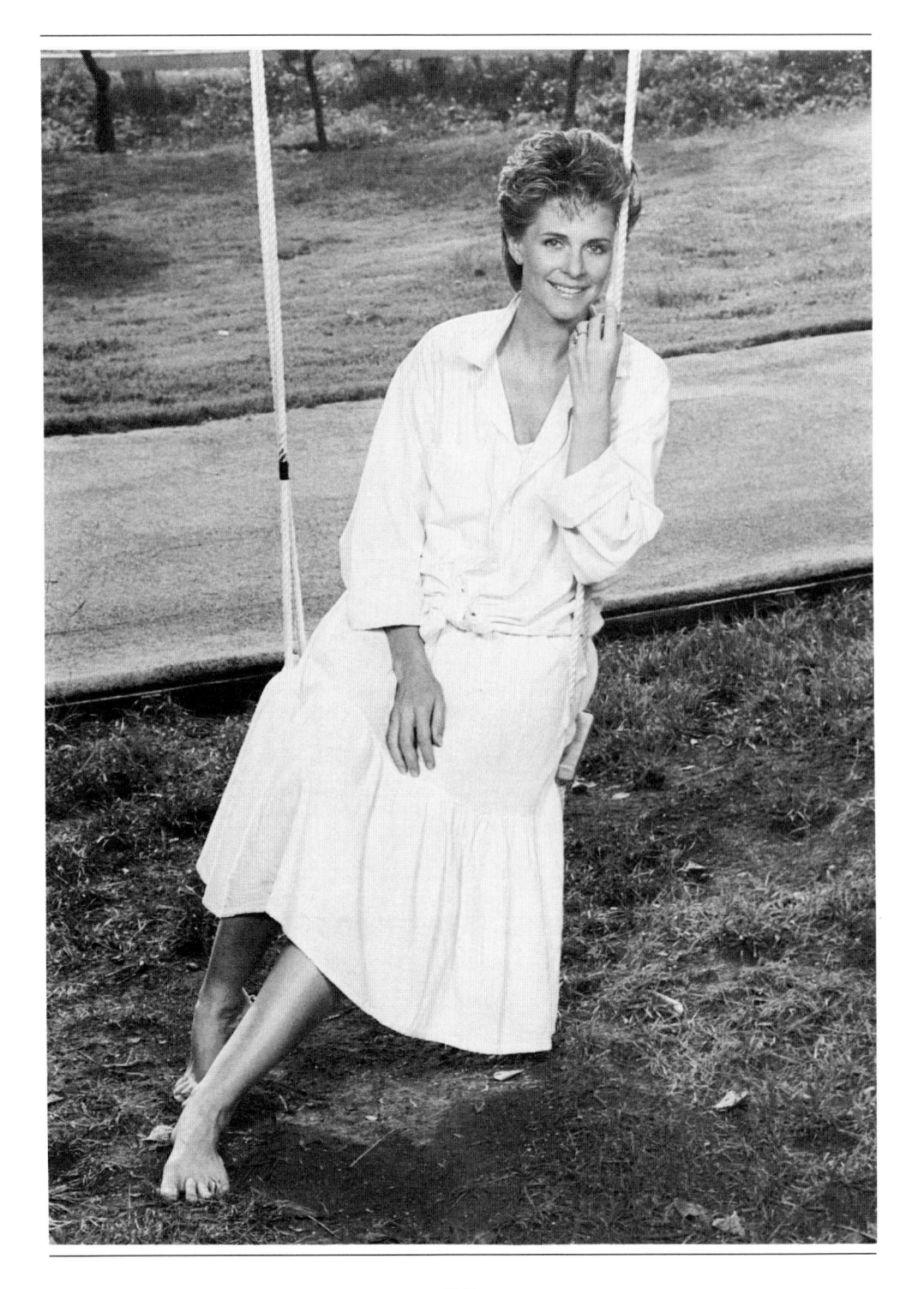

GETTING YOUR BODY AND HEAD BEHIND YOUR FACE

"Beauty is but skin deep" is an old English proverb. But Herbert Spencer, an English philosopher, once said: "The saying that beauty is but skin deep is a skin-deep saying."

I go along with Spencer. Beauty is much more than just what is out there on the surface. Outer appearance is more than a look, a style of painting your eyes or lips. It is a mirror of what's going on inside the body. It shows the world your general health, your inner strength, your contentment, your happiness, or your lack of these qualities.

If you are stressed, you tend to wear the tension right out there on your face. I know I do. I know many a beautiful woman whose face has lost much of the natural appeal because of the stress that protrudes from within.

To me, beauty is a holistic thing, meaning it involves your body and mind and what you do or do not do for them.

I have a total approach to beauty; or rather, the beauty part seems to take care of itself when I take good care of my physical and emotional health.

I would like to share some of my ideas with you. They are the results of years of learning, of growing, of trial and error. These are the things that work for me. They represent an approach that has had a great sustaining effect on me, allowing me to pursue a busy career as an actress, operate a production company, and, last, but far from least, tend to the needs of two young demanding sons.

Outer beauty can be molded, sculpted, and painted. It can be magnified by a camera angle or a mascara brush. But if the foundation beneath is weak, you are in trouble. The beauty will not last.

It is important that you give that foundation—your body—the best possible nourishment you can. That also means eating a nutritious diet. In the next chapter I will tell you how I handle my diet.

More and more health professionals talk about how stress can undermine both physical and mental health. In my life, and perhaps in yours, there is considerable tumult, and so, I have had to find ways to deal with the stress that arises. In the chapter titled "Rest, Relaxation, and Stress," I will share some practical ideas with you about that.

Finally, in the last chapter, I have some thoughts about makeup; the chemicals we apply and take into our bodies and their relationship to health; and the importance of exercise.

I hope you will find some of these ideas helpful.

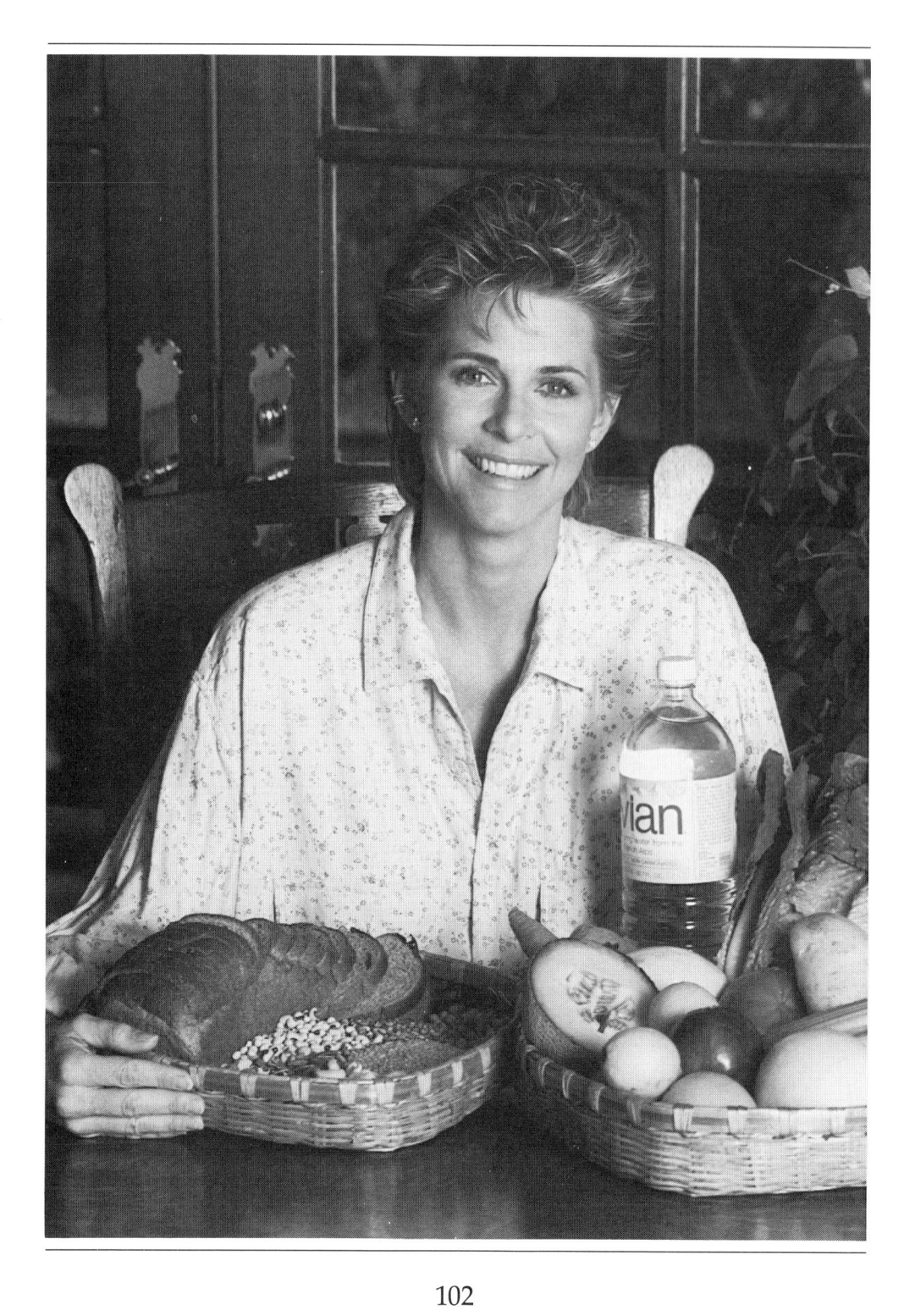

EATING FOR BETTER HEALTH, ENERGY, AND BEAUTY

I eat with purpose. I want every bit of food I put in my mouth to go to work for me: to help create optimal health and to supply my body with the energy it needs to handle the demands of my life-style.

If you eat for health, you are also eating for beauty.

The meals my family and I eat are very simple; they consist of the freshest and most wholesome natural and unprocessed food I can buy. My orientation is to a vegetarian-type diet comprised primarily of complex carbohydrates. That means whole grain cereals, such as brown rice and whole wheat; legumes, such as tofu and beans; fresh vegetables and fruits; and pasta.

I became a vegetarian in the early seventies, after I learned about all the chemicals that were being used to enhance the growth of animals raised for human consumption.

I learned that there are literally thousands of these chemicals. In some cases, the use of a particular chemical in animals has not been approved by the government. Their long-range side effects are not yet known. I was shocked to learn that about half of the antibiotics produced in the United States are injected or supplied to livestock to fatten them up. Recently, I read a congressional subcommittee warning about the "possible significant adverse effects" of these substances, which may be passed on to humans in the meat, milk, and eggs that are consumed.

When we take medication or prescription drugs, we know, for the most part, what we are getting into. At least the doctor or the package warns us of potential side effects. But here we have no idea of what "extras" we are getting with the meat we buy or of the possible harm that may be done to the body.

When I first stopped eating meat, I became concerned that perhaps I wasn't getting enough protein in my diet. I hadn't learned enough yet about nutrition and nonanimal forms of protein, and I was worried that the diet was inadequate to sustain my activities. I was starting to work very hard at the time. So, after about a year and a half of not eating it, I began to add meat back into my diet.

My body had completely adjusted to a vegetarian diet and, to my surprise, I found I couldn't eat beef any more. My body rejected it. Eating meat again made me feel sluggish and not at all well. I felt poisoned. My skin started to break out in strange patches of discoloration. I simply did not work or feel at my best.

I stopped eating red meat altogether. The only meat I would eat from that point on was fish and chicken a few times a week. As I started learning more about food and the value of vegetable protein, even the fish and fowl began to have less importance in my diet. Eventually they disappeared from it entirely.

I have now gone through two pregnancies, delivered healthy babies, and nursed them with no problem at all on what is basically a nonmeat diet. It works wonderfully for me.

THE VALUE OF COMPLEX CARBOHYDRATES

Like me at the beginning, many people balk at the idea of a vegetarian diet, because they are worried about getting enough protein. According to many respected authorities around the world, however, getting enough good protein out of a vegetarian-type diet is no problem, if you eat a wide variety of food.

Dr. U. D. Register, a nutritionist at Loma Linda University in southern California who has studied this question thoroughly for thirty years, maintains that protein is well represented in both quality and quantity in vegetable-source food; even total vegetarians receive an adequate amount.

"If you eat a variety of grains, legumes, and vegetables, there is no problem," he says.

There are different types of vegetarians. Some will eat eggs and dairy; others vegetables alone. In my case, I do eat eggs and dairy, if they belong to a good recipe, but I do not regard them an important part of my diet.

This style of eating represents a low-fat, high-fiber diet that has been scientifically shown to be beneficial for health, growth, and energy. Studies show that vegetarians consume less total fat than people who eat a more typical diet. As a result, they tend to have fewer weight problems and better health.

In recent years more and more athletes, even football players, in fact, are turning from their traditional diets of heavy meat and fat to menus that place a strong emphasis on complex carbohydrates (carbohydrates that come from whole grains, fruits, and vegetables). That is because this type of food delivers the energy they need. One Scandinavian study showed that athletes who went on a high-fat, high-protein diet experienced a big drop in their normal endurance. On a high-carbohydrate vegetarian-type diet, their endurance levels actually doubled.

While I myself am no athlete, I lead a very busy life. I burn a lot of energy. I need efficient food that can supply optimal energy. If I don't get it, I become fatigued. When you are tired, you cannot function well and you don't look well either. It's plain and simple.

Your body needs the starches and natural sugars of carbohydrates; it converts them into glucose, the major fuel for muscular activity. This raw material is the body's fuel.

GOOD VERSUS BAD CARBOHYDRATES

Many people think of carbohydrates as food to avoid. "Makes you fat," they believe.

But it's not the carbohydrate that is the guilty party. The guilty party is you, or the food manufacturer. The crime is what is *done* to the original food, not the food itself. Here's what I mean: A baked potato by itself is only 145 calories. Put two pats of butter on it, however, and you've added 75 calories. French-fried potatoes and potato chips are cooked in oil. Oil is fat and that means calories—twice as much as in carbohydrates. Ten fries are 214 calories. Ten chips are 114. But who stops at ten?

Refined carbohydrates are an example of how food is commercially "adulterated." This group of foods includes white rice, white flour products (cakes, cookies, white bread), and refined white flour, pasta products (not to be confused with pasta made from 100 percent durum wheat semolina, which is a good source of complex carbohydrates and has less than half the calories of white flour pasta), white sugar and sweets, and canned fruits. These items are generally processed to such a degree that they are broken down by the body very quickly. This causes undesirable roller-coaster effects on energy and blood sugar levels.

Refined carbohydrate foods tend to deliver many "empty calories' because of the high amount of white sugar they contain. Donuts and soda are good examples. (You find them all around movie sets, too!) A 12-ounce can of soda contains 9 teaspoons of sugar. A glazed donut has 6.

White sugar is used to sweeten a wide variety of foods because it is cheap to manufacture. Many medical authorities worry that it is being consumed in quantities that are far too large. Believe it or not, the average American eats 7,280 teaspoons of sugar a year, which is quite damaging to health.

White sugar is a refined simple sugar. That means it is rapidly absorbed into the bloodstream and causes the level of glucose to soar. This provides a short-lived burst of energy, usually followed by a pronounced sag in vitality as the body responds by normalizing the glucose level. Along with the energy drop, you may also experience headaches and irritability.

As the name implies, complex carbohydrates contain a more complex type of chemical structure. They release their sugars at a slower and more desirable rate during the digestive process. Moreover, unlike the refined carbohydrates that often come devoid of anything other than calories and vast amounts of chemical additives, these foods contain many vitamins and minerals.

FIBER

Another important reason to choose complex carbohydrates is their superior fiber content. Fiber increases the rate at which waste products are eliminated from the bowels and has, in some cases, been found to decrease the absorption of some sugars and fats. Fiber is even thought to lower blood cholesterol levels in some individuals.

Fiber is the portion of plant foods that human digestive enzymes cannot break down. These fibers are hygroscopic; that is, they absorb moisture, increase in size, and act as a natural laxative. Many medical authorities believe that fiber can help prevent—and perhaps can even be used in the treatment of—colon cancer, diverticulosis, irritable bowel syndrome, and hemorrhoids.

WATER

Water is as important to the body as any food, if not more so. Water is essential to all living things. After all, our bodies are comprised mostly of water and our skin is more than 50 percent water. Our diet should include six to eight glasses each day in addition to any other liquids. Without sufficient water, the body cannot effectively eliminate toxins and other waste materials through the kidneys and colon, and the skin has to work overtime to release them through the pores. When this is the case, the skin loses elasticity, is prone to blemishes, suffers a decreased resistance to injury and infection, and becomes dry. The suppleness and resiliency of the skin must come from within. No amount of moisturizer applied topically can provide the benefits obtained from drinking six to eight glasses of water each day.

MY MENU

In my daily diet, I usually eat only fresh fruit or juice in the mornings—always fresh, nothing from cans. This usually keeps me going until lunchtime.

I find that when I eat solids for breakfast I seem to be a little sluggish afterward. I don't have my usual zip, and I also tend to eat more throughout the day.

Generally, I eat my first solids at midday, earlier or later depending on my schedule. If I have a heavy day, then I will usually have lunch at around 11 A.M.

What I eat for my lunch depends on where I am eating. I most enjoy a combination of whole grains and beans. My favorite dish is brown rice along with a mixture of azŭki and pinto beans.

If no kitchen is available when I am filming on location, I will have these kind of simple dishes prepared for me on a hot plate. It is just what I need. It provides plenty of good protein and usable energy.

In restaurants I can usually get by with a salad and baked potato. I don't eat anything swimming in rich sauces.

Dinner usually involves a serving of some whole grain dish with vegetables or legumes. I like to use lots of tofu (soy bean curd) and nuts in my dishes.

One of the favorite foods in our house, which we eat for lunch and even dinner sometimes, are whole-wheat pancakes. I call them "McNeil's pancakes," after Dr. Jim McNeil, a good friend who created the recipe. For anyone interested in trying it, here it is:

McNEIL'S PANCAKES

1 cup whole-wheat flour	3 tablespoons raw sunflower seeds
1 cup rolled oats	
1 cup bran flakes	1½ teaspoons baking soda
3 eggs	½ teaspoon salt
3 tablespoons wheat germ	2 tablespoons honey
3 tablespoons ground sesame seeds	4 tablespoons safflower oil
	2 cups buttermilk

While combining the ingredients, add water to thin out the rather thick consistency of the batter. Make it much thinner than you would regular pancake batter. Then use either butter or vegetable oil to fry the pancakes.

These pancakes are definitely a great energy booster and are nutritious. When I was nursing my first child and working at the same time, I just could not seem to get enough to eat. I couldn't find anything that really satisfied my hunger for the amount of energy I was putting out. With this dish I found I could go quite a few hours without having to stop and refuel. I normally use either honey or pure maple syrup to sweeten food. When I cook oatmeal or any other cereals, I will sweeten them with bananas or raisins.

My particular diet is the result of trying to educate myself about nutrition over the years and create an eating regimen that works for me. I realize that it is not for everybody and I am not recommending it as any kind of a "Bionic Woman's Diet."

I firmly believe that everyone should learn as much as possible about food and try to find an eating program that fits their needs and life-style. Probably the best thing you can do for yourself is to follow a diet that gives you as much variety as you need, while still providing proper nutrition.

SUPPLEMENTS

I do not believe in going overboard on vitamin and mineral supplements. I take a good quality, medium-potency multivitamin and mineral formula on a daily basis along with a calcium supplement. I feel that megadoses of vitamins are not necessary, unless you are dealing with specific problems that large amounts of vitamins can help.

I do believe, however, that moderate supplementation is useful because of three factors:

- The depleted nature of the soil in which our food is grown
- The further depletion of nutrients during the processing and mass-distribution of food
- The constant drain on our bodies of essential nutrients because of the stressful, fast-paced lives we lead, and the harmful effect of chemicals in our environment

Even if you think you are eating a healthy balanced diet, the extra help from supplementation is probably going to be beneficial. It's good insurance, anyway.

If you eat less than a healthy diet, you should supplement for sure. If you eat regularly in fast-food restaurants, you could be developing deficiencies in a number of important nutrients.

Studies done by the Department of Agriculture and other government agencies repeatedly find many Americans grossly deficient in calcium, iron, zinc, magnesium, and vitamins A, B_1, B_2, B_6, and C.

Following are some of the major nutrients that are related to beauty.

Vitamin A has a lot to do with your skin. You need enough in your diet to have smooth, soft, healthy-looking skin. It is responsible for the integrity of the epithelium, a tightly knit top layer of cells covering every surface of the body, including the skin.

A shortage affects the female cycle and can contribute to excessive menstruation.

If your diet is built on fast foods, be aware that these dishes are notoriously short of vitamin A. In recent years, the medical community has been given growing attention to the cancer protection provided by the vitamin A found in green and yellow vegetables.

Good sources of this vitamin include carrots, sweet potatoes, dark leafy greens, apricots, cantaloupe, and winter squash.

B-complex vitamins also affect your skin. Make sure you are getting enough. Disorders of the skin, hair, nails, and nervous system occur where there is a deficiency of most of the members of this family of vitamins.

For instance, deficiencies of thiamine, riboflavin, biotin—three members of this family—are known to cause scaling and redness of the skin, especially around the mouth and nose.

Vitamin B_6 promotes tanning of the skin. You can get the many benefits of sun without overexposure.

One of the problems with refined carbohydrates is that many of the B-complex vitamins are processed out of them. Whole grain products, brewer's yeast, and liver are the best sources for these important nutrients.

Vitamin C in ample quantity is necessary for the production, formation, and maintenance of good-quality collagen. Collagen is the intercellular protein "cement" that binds tissue throughout the body. It holds together muscles, the blood vessels, the ligaments, tendons, cartilage and skin, giving them all strength and structure. Collagen is also the honeycomb into which minerals are deposited to form bone. Without collagen, a body would become unglued and would collapse. Good-quality collagen, among other things, is important to the skin's support tissue and thereby to elasticity and suppleness.

Vitamin C also seems to play a role in every bodily function and is important in maintaining strong resistance against colds and viruses.

The best sources of this vitamin are fresh—not canned—fruits and vegetables.

Vitamin E helps the heart and red blood cells carry oxygen to all the cells of the body. It offers protection against the damaging effects of many environmental poisons in the air, water, and food.

Vitamin E also seems to play a role in combating premature aging of the skin.

Good sources of this vitamin are cold-pressed vegetable oils, eggs, wheat germ, sweet potatoes, and leafy vegetables.

Calcium is especially important for a woman in order to maintain good bone density. It is one of the few supplements that I take. I find that when taken before bedtime it is a nice relaxant.

Dairy products are the best sources of calcium. Sesame seeds are also high in calcium, and I use a lot of them in my cooking. I will grind up the seeds to a powder and then sprinkle them in dishes.

Zinc is a protector against hair loss and thinning. It is important, too, for the maintenance of good collagen and strong resistance.

This nutrient is grossly deficient in refined foods. Good sources are eggs, liver, soybeans, seeds, and nuts. (See appendixes A and B for other natural sources of vitamins and minerals.)

WHEAT GRASS JUICE FOR THE SKIN

One of my favorite drinks is wheat grass juice. I buy it at the health food store freshly squeezed. Even with all the other things that I do, I feel it makes a good contribution to the suppleness of my skin. It tends to make the wrinkles softer on my face. When I don't have it for a while, I notice my skin becomes just a bit drier.

Wheat grass, when taken in the form of a freshly squeezed juice like this, is a good body cleanser. I try to drink about one ounce a day.

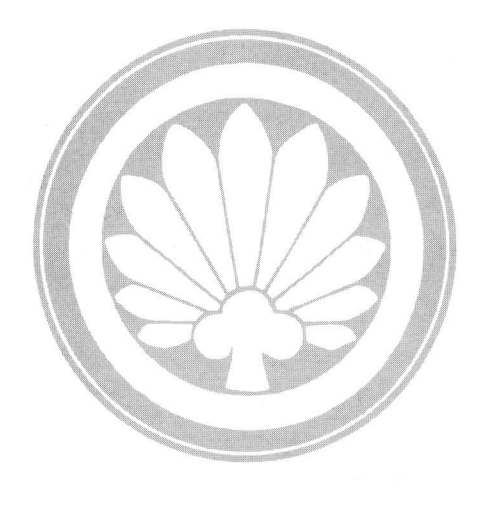

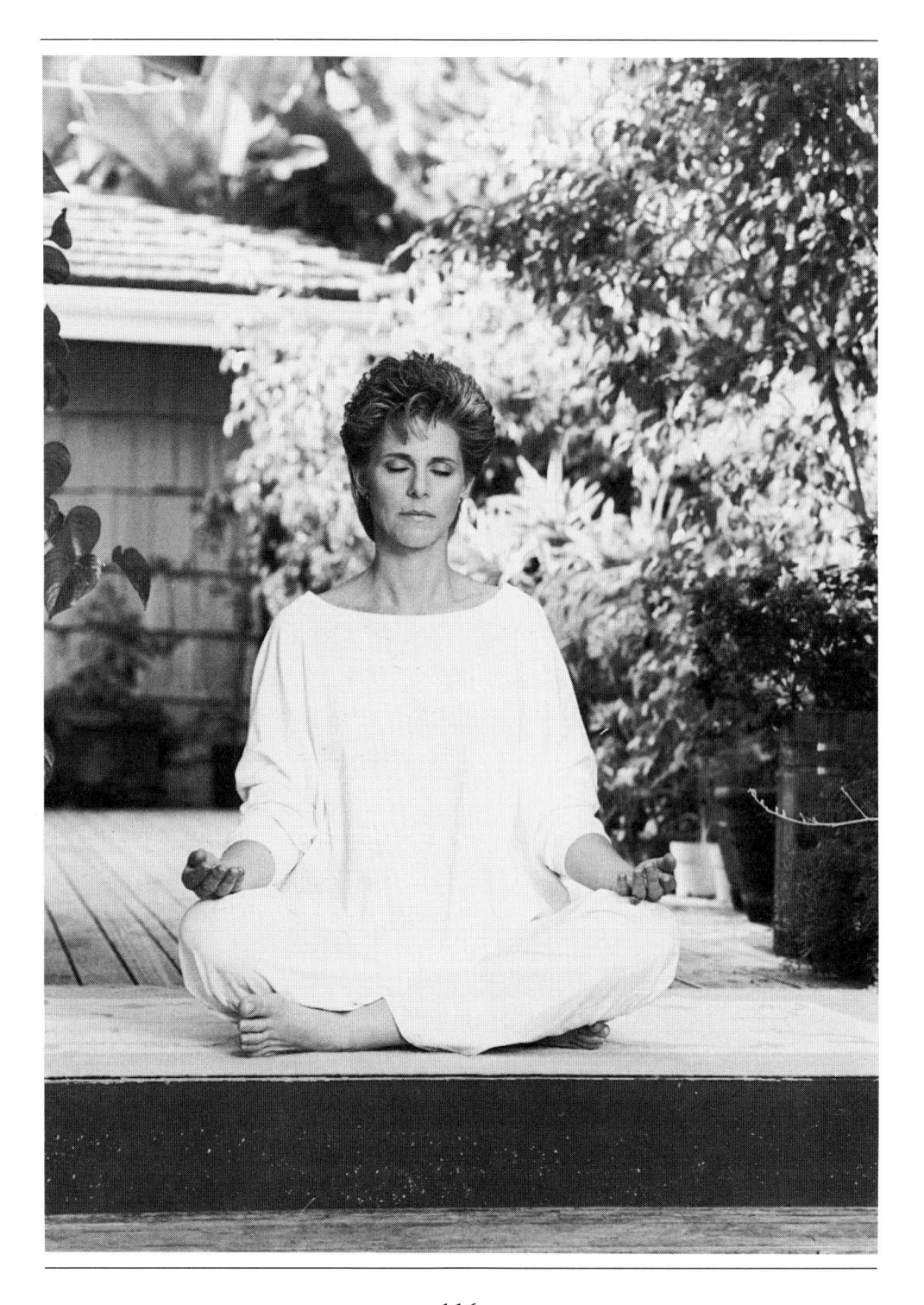

REST, RELAXATION, AND STRESS

During the last five years, people have continually been telling me how good I look, and they want to know what I am doing now that I wasn't doing before. I look better than ever, they say, despite the fact that I have been working harder than ever and that I have become a mother twice during this time.

My only answer to this is that I have been doing more intensive work on myself—internally, I mean. I see to it that I give my body, mind, and spirit the kind of nourishment they need in order for me to function effectively at many demanding levels and still be a sensitive, caring individual.

The kind of nourishment I am talking about here involves not food, but intangibles such as rest and meditation to preserve my tranquility and creative energy in a stressful world.

REST

Everybody has their own individual requirement for sleep, which changes from time to time, depending upon what is going on in his or her life. Sometimes you need more sleep, sometimes less. One person may get by with six hours, the other needs eight.

I have discovered that the more sleep I can get before midnight, the more rested I feel the next day. I make a great effort to be in bed by 9:30 or 10 P.M. That way, when I have to arise early at 4 A.M. or 5 A.M., as I do when I am making a film, I have no problem. I have plenty of energy; I feel extremely good. When I am not filming and I go to bed at, say, 11 P.M. or midnight, even though I can sleep late in the morning, I still never feel as rested as I do when I have gone to bed earlier.

I am no early bird. I am, by nature, a night person, and love staying up late. I had to teach myself to change, but the difference I feel in energy is well worth the effort.

RELAXING AND STRESS

I do a number of things to help me deal with the accumulation of tension and stress in my life. One of those fundamental tools we have already discussed: the massage of facial points in the Acupressure Facelift. This has provided me with a handy way to defuse some of the tension I sometimes develop in my face and jaw; it is also a way to give me a quick infusion of relaxation.

Let me share a few other methods that I find helpful. Perhaps they will be of practical use to you, as well.

DEEP BREATHING

I constantly try to monitor my breathing, particularly in situations of anxiety or stress.

When we get tense, our breathing tends to become shallow and more rapid. That affects the entire body. There is less efficiency. Perception suffers.

When I become aware that this is happening, I consciously slow down my breathing. I will take two, three, four deep breaths. Immediately, I experience a release of tension and stress in my body and mind. I feel more relaxed. My perception of things around me returns to normal.

I use this technique constantly while I am working. It always helps me relax under the intense conditions involved in my work.

I recall a particular situation during the production of a TV movie. There were a couple of crew members who were always arguing and snapping at each other. There was a lot going on in my life at the time, and my emotions were closer to the surface than usual. With this friction around me, it was difficult for me to play this particular character, who was supposed to be full of life, joy, and wonder. To help myself, I left the set frequently for a few minutes at a time. I would go and sit down, then quiet my mind and do some deep breathing. This would enable me to relax quickly. I would return to the set more relaxed, which enabled me to play the part more effectively.

For me, this method restores my natural state of being. That state, not just in me, but in all of us, is a state of happiness. That is our essential energy, but too often it is blocked and throttled by layers of stress and fatigue.

During that film, as in many other working situations, the deep breathing came to my rescue, allowing me to defuse the stress and bring all my skills and needed emotions to bear on the task at hand.

VISUALIZATION

Creating tranquil images in the mind can also be helpful.

Think for instance of a place . . . the prettiest most serene place you can think of . . . your very own special place where nobody else goes. Only you. You can create such a place in your mind and use it to calm yourself whenever you want to work something out or you simply want to be at peace with yourself.

You do not have to sit and do it for hours. All you need to do is take a few minutes, close your eyes, and go to this place. Your body chemistry will shift to a more tranquil mode and you will feel your body and mind relax. It is also helpful if you do the deep breathing along with this.

An effective image to use is a wind-blown lake. In your imagination you calm down the wind and see the ripples become less and less apparent until the water is absolutely still. This imaging has a corresponding effect on your body.

Another variation is to sit in a chair or lie down on your back. With your eyes closed, go through your entire body and see the different parts relaxing. Start at your feet. Then the calves. The knees. The thighs. And so on until you cover all parts. This also has a good, calming effect.

What this all boils down to is taking a few minutes for yourself. We all must, at times, just shut out the world around us and get in touch with our true inner feelings. Sitting quietly alone, we can better sort through our thoughts and make decisions when we are not being bombarded by the very things that cause us to be stressed.

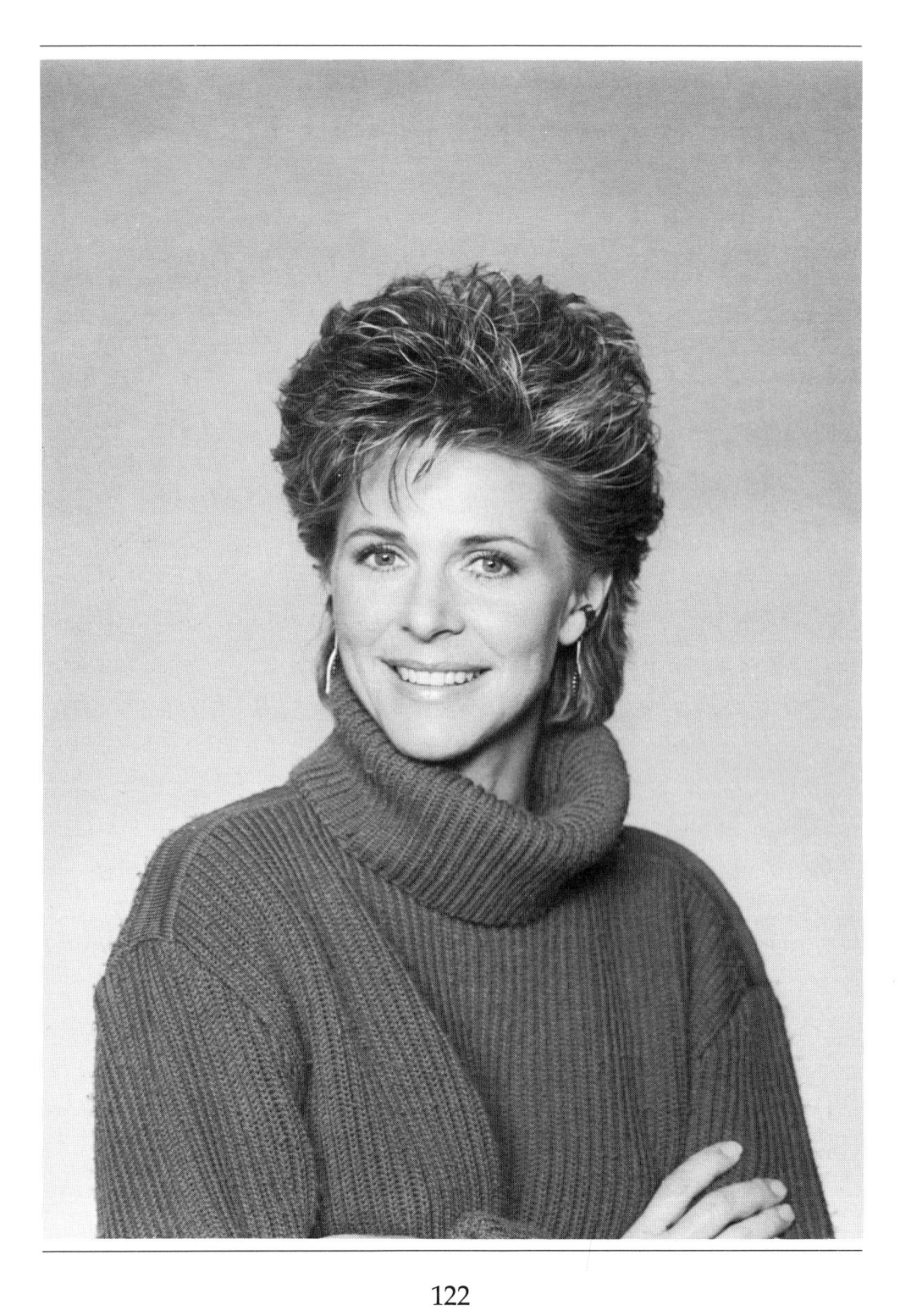

BEAUTY TIPS

When you feel good about yourself and about life, that feeling radiates through your face like sunshine. Whether you are wearing makeup or not isn't important. The feeling comes through. Even the person who is expertly made up is not nearly as attractive or as effective, I think, as the person who is glowing from the inside.

I only wear makeup when I am working in front of the cameras or when I have to make a public appearance. Even in these situations I only use the minimum. My on-camera makeup is extremely minimal for most of the roles I play. Occasionally, when I have a special character role, I may have to use a heavier makeup. But the heaviest I ever use is the equivalent of what most people think of as street makeup. Outside of these occasions, I don't wear any.

I feel that women who do wear heavy makeup all the time, are doing their skin and themselves a disservice. They are creating an artificial look on their face that can create a barrier to natural expressions toward events and people in their life.

I regard makeup as something that should be used sparingly, bits of it here or there to enhance, rather than hide your true appearance. I do not believe that makeup should make you look like something you aren't. And I don't think it is something we should depend upon to make us feel beautiful.

CHEMICAL BEAUTY

We live in a chemical world, and we don't really know what effect all these chemicals have on us. My approach to beauty and personal hygiene products is similar to my approach to food—as natural and with as few chemical additives as possible.

The ingredients lists on many product labels read like a chemical *Who's Who*. Who knows what they are and who knows what they do to the body? I believe in using products only when I can recognize the ingredients on the label.

For instance, some of the so-called beauty soaps contain ingredients that I don't recognize, so I don't use them. I use a balanced glycerine-based beauty soap. It does the job that I need it to do: wash off pollution, dust, and dead skin cells. It doesn't dry my skin, as some of the highly chemicalized beauty soaps tend to do.

Who needs complicated soap? Mechanics and construction workers come home with dirty, grimy skin. They require something special. I don't.

I use an unscented moisturizing cream on my face—unscented because the scents used in beauty and facial products are made of chemicals. The added scent does not help the cream do its job any better.

Chemicals in facial products are absorbed into the skin and who knows what they do or where they go once they are under the skin's surface? Are they causing any subtle problems in the biochemistry of your body?

I hope you don't get the impression that I live in mortal fear of grotesque allergic reactions or chemical intoxication. I simply want to avoid any possible reaction at all. Why should I apply anything to my skin that it doesn't need? Why should I buy something that my body doesn't require? I simply feel the way most people feel: good health is important to me.

In this world we live in it is virtually impossible to escape harmful substances, but we can try to become aware of them and to cut down on our exposure to them.

Have you ever gone into a beauty salon for a treatment and emerged from it feeling punch-drunk, irritable, headachy, fatigued, or confused? If you have, that's probably because you have a sensitivity to one or more of the chemicals added to the products they used.

Sensitivity to cosmetics and toiletries is part of a general susceptibility to chemicals, often of the petroleum-based type; which might indicate a potential for problems from many different sources. Petroleum-based chemicals are incorporated in a vast array of products we use in daily life—soaps, detergents, synthetic fabrics, sprays, newspaper print, alcohol—and, of course, petroleum is at the very heart of the smoggy air many of us breathe.

Some doctors who specialize in these kinds of environmental sensitivities feel that a great many people have difficulties with such chemicals and that the symptoms can manifest themselves in any variety of mental, emotional, or physical ways.

I have learned that reactions often involve the nervous system, resulting in headaches, anxiety, or depression. But anything can be affected, even the diet and a person's tolerance for certain foods.

A doctor I know reports that his after-shave lotion made his daughter itchy and irritable every time he kissed her.

"Her problem, or anybody else's, for that matter," he says, "could be the petroleum-based alcohol used as a carrier in the formula or the scent, which might be made up of forty or fifty different chemicals. Any one chemical could be the sensitizing agent, or any combination of them."

Most scents used in cosmetics and toiletries are clearly far from natural. There are two major ways cosmetics and their chemical constituents can affect the body. One is through direct contact. For the ultra-sensitive individual, applying the wrong cosmetic can be akin to applying poison ivy. The result is a local irritation of the skin, a kind of contact dermatitis.

Airborne scents can also constitute direct contact, striking at sensitive eye, nose, or throat tissue.

Inhalation is the other major route for molecules of an active substance to enter the bloodstream. It is known that a sensitive individual can even develop joint pains after being exposed to the odor of perfume, nail polish, or nail polish remover.

Chemical sensitivities are genuinely individual. One person might be sensitive to perfume A, but not to perfume B. Perfume A contains something that this individual cannot tolerate.

The cause for such sensitivities seems to be highly complex and not totally understood by science. One factor may be the deluge of strange new chemicals in recent years. The human species, which has evolved without these chemicals, simply may not be able to efficiently adapt to them. Some people have more difficulty adapting than others. It depends on the strength of individual tolerance; that is, the way a person's body deals with foreign substances. This strength differs from person to person.

At any rate, this is why I try to cut down the number of chemicals in my own life. We should all think about all the things we put into and on our bodies to make us look and smell better.

One parting tip on this subject: If you think you are sensitive to the chemicals of beautification, schedule your beauty parlor appointments for the beginning of the week. Try to be the first appointment on Monday. That way there is a minimum of chemical exposure. The shop was closed on Sunday. The place will have aired out. If you go on Friday afternoon or Saturday, you may be inviting trouble.

SMOKING

You have probably heard a million times by now how bad smoking is for your health. I will add to that: Anything that is bad for your health also cannot be good for your beauty.

As a teenager, I was a pack-a-day smoker. I remember the dry and pale skin, to say nothing of the way my hair and clothes smelled. It is now known that smoking constricts the blood vessels, impairing the natural flow of blood and oxygen and nutrition. After I stopped smoking, I soon noticed an improvement in my skin, among other things.

Scientists have long known that heavy smoking deprives all the tissues of the body, especially the skin, from needed oxygen; it constricts the blood vessels that carry the oxygen. Simply put, skin not receiving its fair share of oxygen will shrivel, wrinkle, and age at a faster pace.

In one medical study, the researchers suggested that heavy smoking could make a person look as much as twenty years older.

ALCOHOL AND DRUGS

I think that people get very old very fast from this kind of activity. Depending on which drug is involved, there are various destructive processes generated throughout the body.

If you care about your outer beauty and your inner strength, if you really care about yourself and the people who love you, this is definitely not the way to go. When I lecture to young women on health, I emphasize this point.

Many years ago, before I became interested in holistic medicine and spiritual growth, I was like many people of my age. Drinking and smoking were the things to do.

On the surface level I found there was a direct negative effect. There were dark circles under my eyes that makeup never seemed to cover. But skin and appearance are really the least of the problems.

Dependence brings people to a state where they don't have the inner strength to accomplish what they need or want to do in life. Those who need a push in some way will rely more and more on stimulants; those who want to block out things will rely on depressants. The whole aspect or quality of inner beauty, where your own personal glow comes through to animate and enhance the surface, all that just goes by the wayside. Drugs are not an answer to anything.

EXERCISE

Exercise certainly is important in maintaining an attractive appearance as well as contributing in many ways to general health. I see another important value in exercise: enhancing relaxation and eliminating physical and mental stress, allowing you to project a natural state of being.

I do a twenty-to-thirty minute series of formal movements that emphasize breathing and stretching. The routine is called "psychocalisthenics," and it was developed by Oscar Ichazo, the founder of Arica, a New York–based human-growth movement. (For more information, contact the Arica Institute, 150 Fifth Avenue, #912, New York, NY 10011, Tel.: 212-807-9600.)

This activity is sometimes called "yoga in motion." It looks something like dance or *T'ai Chi*. It works every muscle in your body, provides aerobic benefits, and, in general, is the most well-rounded program that I know of. It is the first exercise routine I have been able to stick to in my life! I had been known to drive to my mailbox!

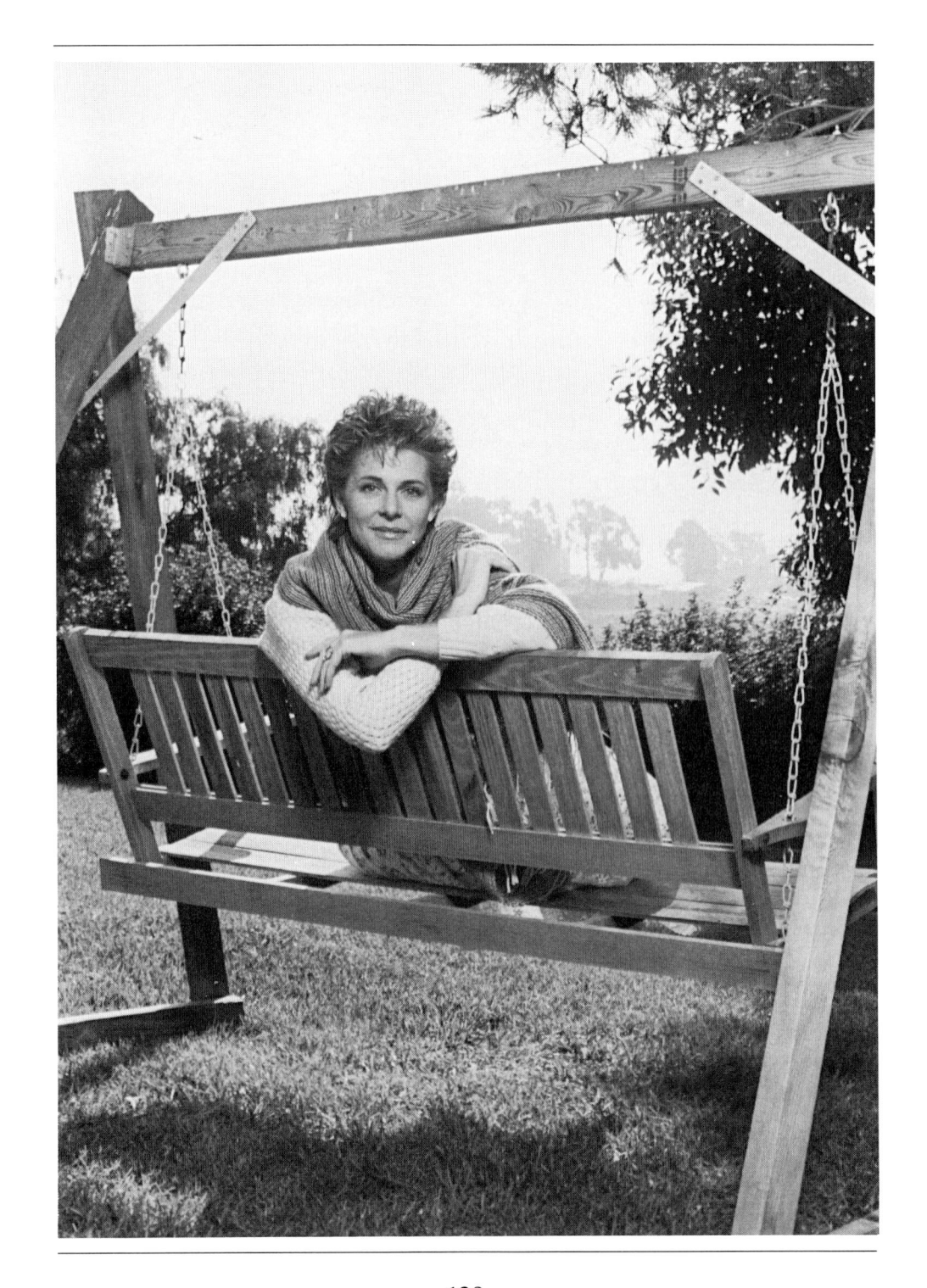

SOME PARTING WORDS

The new beauty is not really so new. The ancient Chinese and writers throughout the centuries have known that beauty is more than outward appearance, that it must come from within. Beauty reflects your inner well-being—your physical and spiritual health.

The Acupressure Facelift is a tool that you now have to make the most of your looks. By following the program I have outlined, you can soften and sometimes eliminate facial wrinkles, and keep new ones from appearing. It is a simple, relaxing method that you can easily integrate into your busy daily schedule. You will notice changes almost immediately, and a simple maintenance program will ensure that the changes are permanent.

The Acupressure Facelift will stimulate your energy to make you more health conscious. I have also told you about the things that help me maintain good health and skin tone. I hope you will use these tips to design a program of diet and exercise for yourself. There are also many helpful books on the market that you can use. Ask your doctor to help you choose the foods that make up a balanced diet.

All of our organs must function at their optimal level if we are to be in the best of health. The skin is the body's largest organ and we have to look at it all the time. Its functions are impaired when the other organs, and when the body as a whole, are not properly nourished. There is no reason why we all cannot renew our beauty and have flawless complexions, firm bodies, and good health.

PART IV

APPENDIXES

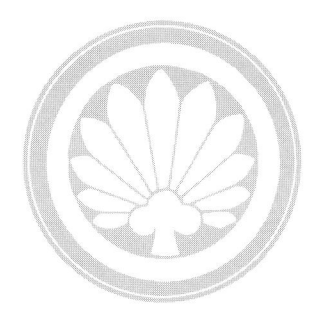

APPENDIX A: VITAMINS

This appendix lists the three vitamins most beneficial to the skin and the foods in which these vitamins can be found. (Read top to bottom, column by column—the foods are listed in order of highest in vitamin content.)

VITAMIN A

Hot red pepper
Dandelion greens
Sorrel
Carrot
Dried apricot
Kale
Spinach
Collard greens
Cress
Sweet potato
Parsley
Turnip greens
Turnip
Mustard greens
Swiss chard
Chives

Watercress
Mango
Sweet red pepper
New Zealand spinach
Dried peach
Winter squash
Fennel
Cantaloupe
Endive
Fresh apricot
Broccoli
Green onion
Loose-leaf lettuce
Papaya
Nectarine
Dried prune

Pumpkin
Fresh peach
Boston/Bibb lettuce
Asparagus
Tomato
Soybean

Watermelon
Orange
Tangerine
Sweet corn
Iceberg lettuce

VITAMIN B$_2$ (RIBOFLAVIN)

Hot red pepper
Almonds
Wheat germ
Wild rice
Mushroom
Turnip greens
Dried chestnut
Millet
Wheat bran
Kelp
Collard greens
Soybeans
Cress
Dandelion greens
Parsley
Cashews
Sesame seeds

Sunflower seeds
Pine nuts
Broccoli
Sorrel
Okra
Dried mung beans
Dried pinto beans
Avocado
Asparagus
Spinach
Dried peach
Pumpkin seeds
Dried pear
Swiss chard
Chives
Peanut
Sweet corn

VITAMIN C

Acerola cherries
Guava
Sweet red pepper
Kale
Parsley
Collard greens
Orange peel
Turnip greens
Sweet green pepper
Sorrel
Broccoli
Brussel sprouts
Horseradish
Watercress
Cauliflower
Lemon with peel
Orange with peel
Cress
Persimmons
Kohlrabi
Red cabbage
Strawberries
Chives
Papaya
Savoy cabbage

Peeled lemon
Spinach
Peeled orange
Orange juice
Common cabbage
Lemon juice
Grapefruit juice
Lime
Turnip
Mango
Dandelion greens
Gooseberries
Cantaloupe
Asparagus
Lime juice
Green onion
Oriental radish
Tangerine
Fennel
Okra
New Zealand spinach
Breadfruit
Lima beans
Soybean
Onion

APPENDIX B: MINERALS

Listed below are those minerals most beneficial to the skin and the foods in which they can be found. (Listed in order of highest in mineral content.)

CARBON

- Nuts
- Olives
- Avocado

CALCIUM

- Sesame seeds
- Seaweed
- Green vegetable leaves
- Almonds
- Sunflower seeds
- Kelp
- Kale
- Parsley
- Orange peel
- Pistachio nuts
- Broccoli
- Fennel
- Lentils
- Rice
- Dried apricot
- Soybean
- Horseradish

POTASSIUM

Kelp	Almonds
Irish moss	Raisins
Soybean	Parsley
Lima beans	Sesame seeds
Rice bran	Dried prunes
Banana	Peanuts
Hot red pepper	Dates
Mung beans	Avocado
Peas	Yam
Dried apricot	Horseradish
Pistachio nuts	Garlic
Dried peach	Millet
Sunflower seeds	Mushroom

FLUORINE

Almonds	Turnip greens
Carrot	Dandelion greens
Beet greens	Spinach

SILICON

- Boston/Bibb lettuce
- Iceberg lettuce
- Parsnip
- Asparagus
- Dandelion greens
- Rice bran
- Horseradish
- Onion
- Spinach
- Cucumber
- Strawberries
- Leeks
- Sunflower seeds
- Artichoke
- Swiss chard
- Loose-leaf lettuce
- Pumpkin
- Celery
- Rhubarb
- Cauliflower
- Cherries
- Apricot
- Dried fig
- Beet
- Tomato
- Carrot
- Watermelon
- Millet
- Apple
- Sweet potato
- Turnip
- Green peas
- Common cabbage
- Radish
- Dried prune
- Potato
- Banana

APPENDIX C: FOOD COMBINATIONS

The following is a chart of food combinations that will let you get the most out of the food you eat. Proper diet is not only what you eat—it's also how and when you eat. You miss out on vital nutrients when you combine foods that digest at different rates.

You will notice that melons do not appear on this chart. This is because they digest at a different rate than all other foods and should be eaten alone, either one hour before or after eating anything else.

Like every other organ in the body, our skin has specific nutritional needs. It reflects what is going on inside. A glowing complexion tells the world that we are in good health.

STARCHES
potato
yam
chestnuts
winter squash
grains
pumpkin
corn
carrot

SWEET FRUITS
banana
date
persimmon
fig

SUB-ACID FRUITS
apple
pear
apricot
cherry
grape
plum
mango
nectarine
berry
peach
loquat
papaya

ACID FRUITS
orange
grapefruit
pineapple
pomegranate
lemon
lime
tomato
grapes

PROTEINS
nuts
seeds
peanuts
dried peas
dried beans
meat
fish

GREEN VEGETABLES

AVOCADO

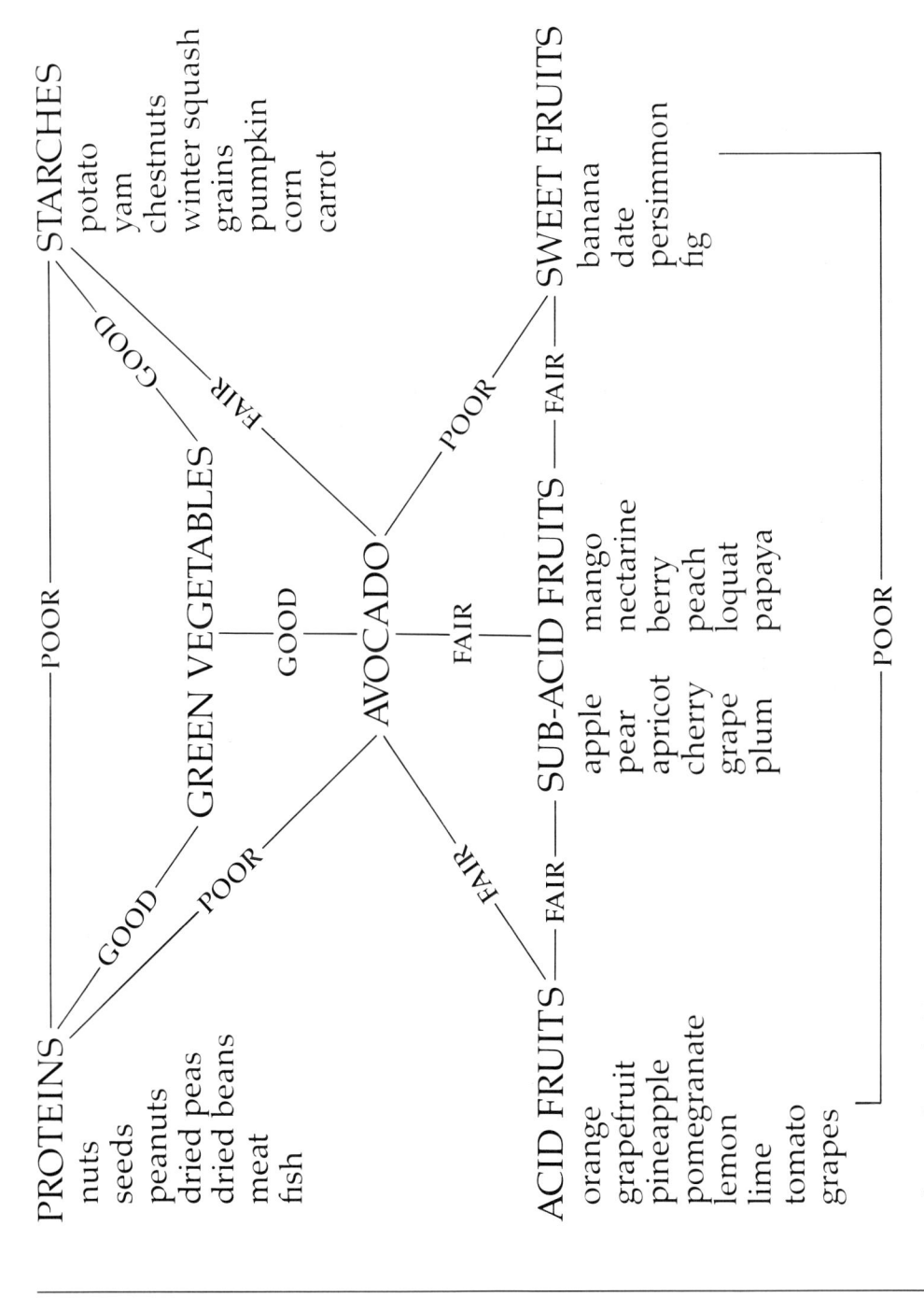

PROTEINS — POOR — STARCHES
PROTEINS — GOOD — GREEN VEGETABLES
STARCHES — GOOD — GREEN VEGETABLES
STARCHES — FAIR — AVOCADO
GREEN VEGETABLES — GOOD — AVOCADO
AVOCADO — POOR — SWEET FRUITS
AVOCADO — FAIR — SUB-ACID FRUITS
SUB-ACID FRUITS — FAIR — SWEET FRUITS
SUB-ACID FRUITS — FAIR — ACID FRUITS
ACID FRUITS — POOR — SWEET FRUITS
ACID FRUITS — POOR — GREEN VEGETABLES
PROTEINS — GOOD — ACID FRUITS (FAIR to AVOCADO)

Source: Compiled by Robert M. Klein.

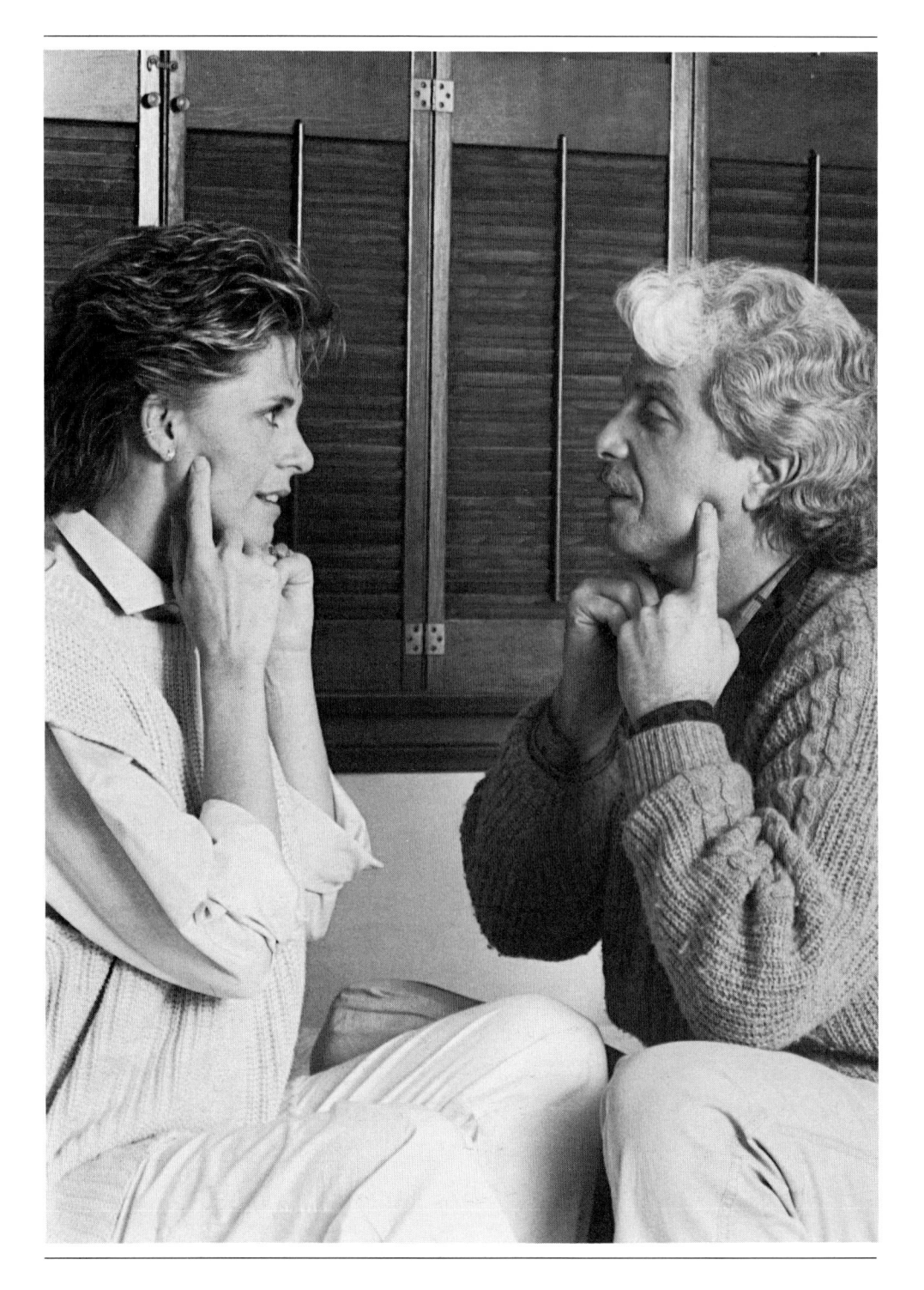

ABOUT THE AUTHORS

LINDSAY WAGNER has endeared herself to both critics and the public alike as one of the most popular actresses of this era. Her career began with a guest shot on "Marcus Welby, M.D." in the early 1970s. Soon after, she parlayed an appearance on "The Six Million Dollar Man" into her Emmy-winning role as "The Bionic Woman," a popular series that ran from 1975 to 1978. She has starred in more than twenty projects during the past several years ranging from motion pictures, television series, mini-series, and television movies. She has portrayed social workers, parents, ambitious career women, mistresses, a death-row murderer, a country doctor, and an amnesia victim, among others. But her criterion has never been the role, but the overall message the film conveys to the viewing public. Her most notable credits include *The Paper Chase, Scruples, Callie & Son, Passions, Child's Cry, I Want to Live, The Incredible Journey of Dr. Meg Laurel, The Two Worlds of Jenny Logan,* and *Memories Never Die.* Today, Lindsay Wagner is exercising her belief in the need for quality television not only as an actress but also as a producer with her own production company. Both on the screen as well as off, Lindsay has championed issues such as preventing child abuse and promoting greater public understanding about learning disabilities and holistic health. When not working in Los Angeles, Lindsay and her two sons enjoy the quiet mountain life outside Portland, Oregon.

ROBERT M. KLEIN is a nutritionist, herbalist, and homeopath, as well as being trained in classical Chinese acupuncture. He was formerly the president of the East-West Acupuncture Society and a director of public information for the National Acupuncture Association. In addition to his health practice, he is currently involved in the development and production of films and videotapes in health-related and other fields.